GYM
SURVIVAL GUIDE

Your Road Map to Fearless Fitness

Gregg Cook & Fatima d'Almeida-Cook

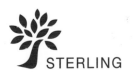

STERLING

New York / London
www.sterlingpublishing.com

GYM SURVIVAL GUIDE

STERLING and the distinctive Sterling logo are registered trademarks of
Sterling Publishing Co., Inc.

Library of Congress Cataloging-in-Publication Data available

10 9 8 7 6 5 4 3 2 1

Published by Sterling Publishing Co., Inc.
387 Park Avenue South, New York, NY 10016
© 2008 by Gregg Cook and Fatima d'Almeida-Cook
Distributed in Canada by Sterling Publishing
C/o Canadian Manda Group, 165 Dufferin Street
Toronto, Ontario, Canada M6K 3H6
Distributed in the United Kingdom by GMC Distribution Services
Castle Place, 166 High Street, Lewes, East Sussex, England BN7 1XU
Distributed in Australia by Capricorn Link (Australia) Pty. Ltd.
P.O. Box 704, Windsor, NSW 2756, Australia

Illustrations: Robin Williams
Book design and layout: Solid Design, Inc.

Printed in China.

Sterling ISBN-13: 978-1-4027-3021-4
        ISBN-10: 1-4027-3021-7

For information about custom editions, special sales, premium and
corporate purchases, please contact Sterling Special Sales
Department at 800-805-5489 or specialsales@sterlingpublishing.com.

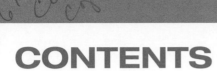

CONTENTS

CONTENTS

CONTENTS

6 THE QUICK START 180

CONTENTS

7 THE CODE OF GYM CONDUCT 216

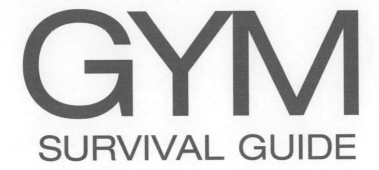

GYM
SURVIVAL GUIDE

INTRODUCTION

The smallest change in perspective can transform a life. What tiny attitude adjustment might turn your world around?

OPRAH WINFREY

THE GYM is a unique world. It's a wonderland where new and exciting experiences beckon from around every corner—dozens of classes to try, machines galore, pools, tracks, treadmills. You can start with the StairMaster, or head to the pool for some Aqua Aerobics. Do you want to try squatting at the Smith machine, or how about some spinning with the cyclists? Have you heard about the bouncing that goes on in the Rebound class? Maybe you'd rather try sparring with the boxers or give Cardio Kickboxing a shot. There's also Capoeira, Yoga, Pilates, BOSU, Gyrotonics, Gliding, Jump Rope classes, and more machines—Elliptical Trainers, rowing machines, VersaClimbers.

Okay, so you get the idea. If you're new to the Gym Universe, the first thing to realize is that you've got options—lots and lots of options. And it's absolutely okay to feel a little overwhelmed by all of these choices, especially if you don't recognize some of the classes we mentioned above. The gym is a new environment to you, and as with anything new, it's going to take a little time and some getting used to before you feel completely at ease.

DURING your first few visits, you'll have a lot to take in and may find that some run-of-the-mill gym behaviors seem a little bit odd. You'll see people running in place like hamsters on wheels, others repetitively lifting and lowering heavy objects, and still others sitting and standing on what appear to be invisible chairs. In one room, groups of 20 to 40 people prepare for combat, and in another they contort their bodies into forms that resemble braided challah bread.

But don't be too concerned. The Gym Universe won't seem so mysterious once its secrets have been revealed to you. And that's what we're here to do. We have answers for you. Answers and information to help make your early gym experiences as positive and rewarding as we know they can be. With the help of this book, soon you'll have the confidence and the knowledge to move around the place like any other pro.

Welcome to your key to surviving the Gym Universe.

THE LOWDOWN

DON'T WAIT FOR WEIGHT

"I should lose weight before I start working out." We hear this all the time. "I'll get to the gym once I lose some weight." This idea stems from a combination of two things. One is being too embarrassed with your physical appearance to show up at the gym. The other is thinking that working out will make you look bulkier. Both excuses are thoroughly ineffective in helping your cause. A big part of losing weight, if that is your goal, is embarking on a journey toward a more physically active lifestyle. And the sooner you start on that journey, the sooner you'll start seeing results—more energy, increased confidence, and a slimmer physique. As for the idea that working out will make you look bigger or bulkier, it's completely false. Exercise helps you slim down by boosting your calorie burn and increasing your metabolism.

YOUR ROADMAP TO THE GYM UNIVERSE

Here's an outline of how the chapters are arranged and what you can expect to find in each.

Before you begin searching for a gym, you need to know when to look for. Chapter 1, "The Investigation,"—examines types of gym memberships that are available—your very own guide to shopping for a gym. We will go over what to be on the lookout for, questions to ask before agreeing to anything, and how to go about negotiating a good deal.

What are your goals? Are you trying to change something about your life? What do you expect to gain—or lose—by joining a gym? Sometimes, our motivations for wanting to change are not readily apparent to us. Chapter 2, "Goals: The Nuts and Bolts," will give you the tools you need to identify your goals and put them into perspective. We'll help you determine objectives that are obtainable and delineate clear steps you can take to actualize them.

An average gym facility is organized to focus on the essential components of a well-rounded fitness program—resistance training, cardiovascular training, core strength, and flexibility. Chapter 3, "Pieces of the Gym Puzzle," is a guided tour of these parts. It will plot out the different areas of a gym, describing their functions and importance.

Chapter 4, "Group Fitness Classes," is a detailed synopsis of some of the most prevalent and popular classes. It will give you the information you need to be able to walk into any class confidently. Chapter 5, "The Equipment," examines the most common equipment you can expect to find in a gym. We explain the functions and features of each piece of equipment and provide photographs of many of the machines you can expect to use, so you can easily identify them.

Chapter 6, "The Quick Start," is like a free training session, explaining how to use basic pieces of equipment. In Chapter 7, "The Code of Gym Conduct," we will act as your personal gym stylist, providing dress code guidelines and tips to help avoid committing acts of disorderly gym behavior. We've included a Glossary at the end of the book for you to use as a quick reference if you need to look up the definitions of important gym-specific and general fitness vernacular.

We guarantee that after reading the *Gym Survival Guide*, your maiden voyage through gym waters will be nothing but smooth sailing.

Physical fitness is the basis for all other forms of excellence.

JOHN F. KENNEDY

YOU'RE ON YOUR WAY

First of all, congratulations are in order. If you're looking at this book, you're probably thinking of joining a gym or have recently joined one. The decision to lead a healthy and active life is truly the first step to becoming fit. The second step is to show up and do the work. Fitness is a journey, a lifestyle, and those who are in great shape work at it consistently.

The initial intimidation associated with joining a gym, just like trying anything new, will subside as soon as you familiarize yourself with your surroundings. Don't worry about the well-adjusted gym folks around you. They are there for the same reasons you are. They are paying attention to their own workouts, striving for their own results. You fit in. You belong just as much as the guy lifting the massive dumbbell beside you. You deserve to be healthy and fit.

Here's the truth of the matter. Whether you realize it or not, the reason for joining a gym boils down to one simple thing: We all want to feel better. The process of working toward our goals can be an enjoyable one in and of itself. In other

THE LOWDOWN

THE MERITS OF A MASSAGE
Allow yourself to indulge in a massage. We all love a good rubdown and acknowledge its soothing and relaxing effects, but the virtues of a massage go well beyond the feel-good factor. A massage will facilitate the transport of oxygen and nutrients to cells and tissues, accelerating the removal of metabolic waste products from the muscles. A preworkout massage helps warm muscles and prepares them for the exercise that follows; a postworkout massage can alleviate soreness and stiffness and reduce muscle fatigue.

words, the time you spend at the gym should be gratifying and positive all around. Take advantage of everything your gym has to offer. Try every class and every piece of equipment. Be sure to schedule time for the sauna or steam room. Get a massage. Look forward to going to the gym. Keep yourself inspired and motivated. Don't be afraid of trying new things. You never know if you are going to enjoy something until you actually try it. You may surprise yourself.

OUR PHILOSOPHY

So, why do we work out? Why do we voluntarily pepper our already overbooked schedules with physically demanding exercise programs? Aren't our lives already so replete with unwarranted aggravations? What makes working out worthy of our time? Although there are innumerable answers to such questions, below are a few of our favorites in order of increasing significance.

We do it for vanity. It's no mystery— we all want to look good. Incorporating regular workouts into your lifestyle will help you build muscle and burn calories more quickly. Each and every workout brings you closer to your fitness goals, and to a slimmer, trimmer you.

We want to be stronger and healthier. Being stronger in your workouts translates into being stronger in your life: being able to pick up a bag of groceries or your five-year-old child, to walk quickly that extra distance in the airport or mall, to tote that suitcase or papers on a business trip, and so on. You will be a frustrating thorn in the side of aging and its relentless attempts to slow you down. Mattresses overstuffed with cash and international fame and popularity will be of no use to you if you are physically overwrought with too many aches and pains to enjoy them. By working out, you will earn the benefits of stronger muscles, including the most important muscle of all, your heart, and as a result will lessen the chance of developing coronary heart disease. Your joints will be well supported, and your posture will be improved. You will have strong bones, decrease the risk of osteoporosis, increase your metabolism and calorie burning during resistance training, and all in all, increase fat loss. You will be able to function more freely and independently in life, and experience less discomfort well into your golden years.

We do whatever it takes to look good in order to feel good, in an attempt to move toward being happy. Ultimately, the most important answer lies in the fact that our minds, bodies, and spirits are completely interwoven. The secret is this: What you possess becomes unimportant if the path to attaining that possession is unearned. This is true of anything in life. The act of taking control of your body, and working toward becoming stronger, leaner, and healthier overall, will bring results that are valuable psychologically, emotionally, and physically. What makes life worthwhile is actually experiencing it. In the same sense, experience your body and its phenomenal ability to move.

Being fit is your choice, absolutely. A constant one. Only you have the power to choose to make the most of your body. Choose to challenge it. Always choose to treat it right and allow it to become the best body it can possibly be.

THE INVESTIGATION

1

People often say that motivation doesn't last. Well, neither does bathing—that is why we recommend it daily.

ZIG ZIGLAR

THERE ARE several different types of gyms out there, and choosing one that is right for you can make or break your inaugural gym experience. It's a personal decision, so spend some quality time researching your options. Consider your specific needs and preferences, your expectations, and, of course, how much you are willing to spend. You don't want to end up with a membership to a gym that doesn't suit your personality and fitness goals, so put some extra effort into the exploratory process to avoid such a situation. We're here to help guide you every step of the way.

THINGS TO CONSIDER

What are the facility's hours of operation? Do those hours work with your schedule? If you're a 9-to-5er and your gym is only open from 9 a.m. to 6 p.m., you'll never be able to get there and use the facilities during the hours of operation.

Where is the gym situated? Is the location convenient for you? If you know that after a long day's work you'll need to get back in your car and drive 45 minutes just to waltz through the revolving glass doors of the gym, the odds are that your motivation for working out will falter. Now imagine that same drive in bad weather. You're even less likely to make the trek. If you're feeling tired, have worked all day long, and planned on taking an evening spin class, you have the entire long drive's time to convince yourself to skip the class and go out for a couple of margaritas with friends or stop at the donut shop for a comforting snack. A convenient location will limit the opportunity for excuses.

How about a trial run? Most gyms will offer you complimentary access to their facilities for periods ranging from a day to over a week. Here is your golden opportunity to observe and really get a feel for the place. What is the general personality of the gym? How friendly and helpful is the front desk staff? Are the trainers knowledgeable? Who are you surrounded by? Do the members look

happy to be where they are? Ask around. Do members look like they are all competitive bodybuilders? If serious weight training isn't one of your fitness goals, this may not be the right place for you. Are other members predominantly of a specific gender? Will this gender makeup mean that working out will be uncomfortable for you? Have people been members for a long time? If the gym has been around for a while but all the members are new, that's a red flag. How clean is the place? Does the staff return free weights and plates where they belong and keep the place in order?

FIT TIP

MONDAY NIGHT MADNESS

During your trial membership, be sure to visit the gym on a Monday night. This time is typically a gym's busiest. Keep an eye on how crowded it gets. Are people waiting around for a long time to get a free treadmill or to use the squat rack? Is spotting an unoccupied piece of equipment a formidable task? These are all telltale signs of congestion. And congestion means less personal attention, and a lot of loafing around waiting for equipment and floor space.

WHAT YOU WILL FIND

So, what are your options? There are many out there, and they mainly differ in two ways. The gym's frill factor is one. The gym's focus is another. Some gyms have the latest and most high-tech equipment and spa services meant to address every fitness goal. Others have cardio equipment and weight training equipment but offer no group fitness classes. Some facilities focus only on weight training while others offer only a specific genre of classes. Perhaps you know that you respond well to group fitness classes. (Hint: that's a great way to get started if you're a gym fledgling.) Make sure that the gym you join offers a variety of classes at times that will work for you. If you're considering hiring a personal trainer, make sure your gym has a full staff of well-experienced and certified trainers.

FULL-SERVICE GYM

GLAMOUR LEVEL

By "glamour" we mean that these gyms are usually open every day or almost every day of the week, from before the crack of dawn to the witching hours of the night. They provide enough services to doll you up from head to toe—inside and out—and offer a diverse range of classes, personal training, sports-specific training, rehabilitation centers, and nutritional counseling. Some of these gyms also have rock climbing walls, swimming pools, saunas, steam rooms, and spas that will manicure your fingers, pedicure your toes, and knead out all your knots. In the locker rooms you'll find all of the potions and lotions required for comfortable, even luxurious grooming (shampoos, moisturizers, mouthwash, cotton swabs, deodorant, and the like). Many facilities even offer child care so that if your babysitter gets stuck in traffic or has a personal emergency, you can still get in your workout.

Glamour facilities are opulent and wonderful—and will cost you about as much as a small private island off the coast of the Mediterranean. Perhaps you need these extra amenities to trick yourself into actually going to the gym. Rewarding yourself with a manicure-pedicure after a tough workout may be exactly the type of motivation you need. There is absolutely nothing wrong with that, especially if you can afford it. If you can't, this is not an excuse not to become fit. The primping, although fun, is not an essential part of working out and won't get you in shape any more quickly.

BASIC LEVEL

The hours of operation of the more basic full-service gyms are usually comparable with those of glamour-type facilities. Basic fitness centers provide all the equipment you need, both cardio and otherwise, a broad selection of group fitness classes, and perhaps a few extra amenities in the locker rooms, such as shared hair dryers. Some of these gyms also have child-care services available. Basic full-service facilities offer a good selection of services, but without the bells and whistles provided by full-service glamour facilities. If you're looking to get in shape without giving your wallet too much of a workout, a membership to a basic full-service gym is good option for you.

FIT TIP

NICE, BUT NOT NECESSARY

The difference between a glamour gym and a basic one is the difference between having a bed skirt on your bed and not. What is a bed skirt, anyway? Not having one should have no bearing on the overall quality of your sleep. Is it a nice thing to have? Sure, if for nothing else than to hide all the stuff stored underneath the bed. Is it necessary? No.

LIMITED FOCUS GYM

Money talk aside, it's important to consider a facility's approach to fitness. Not every gym offers the full gamut of equipment, classes, and services. Many specialize in one thing or another. Here are some of the most common types you may encounter.

EQUIPMENT FOCUS

Gyms that focus on equipment are fully loaded with strength training and cardio apparatus, but they offer no group fitness classes. This type of facility is great for those who are self-motivated and do not need the variety, guidance, or inspiration group fitness classes usually offer. On-staff trainers often roam around the gym floor looking out for people in need of assistance, so you won't be left to fend for yourself completely should you choose not to hire a personal trainer.

Don't think twice about asking for help with setup or pointers on technique—remembering there is no such thing as a bad question.

An equipment-focus facility is also perfect for what we like to call a "celebrity-style" workout. If you prefer to get in, do your thing by yourself or with your trainer or training partner, and get out with no further fuss or ado, this type of place may be right for you.

THE INVESTIGATION

These kinds of gyms can vary significantly in terms of spa services, locker room amenities, and other frill factors; therefore, they can differ greatly in price as well. Generally, they are less pricey than a full-service gym.

SPECIALIZED CLASS FOCUS

If you are attracted to a specific type of training, you may want to look into a studio that specializes in your area of interest. Yoga, Pilates, gyrotonics, dance, and boxing studios often operate this way. In specialized focus gyms, several classes involving various types and levels of training within your specific interest are scheduled throughout the day. Whether you're a novice, are moderately experienced, or are a pro in your activity of choice, you should be able to find classes that suit your needs and help take you to the next level.

You'll find that joining a class-based studio has wonderful benefits. The instructors at these studios are usually extremely skilled in their fields: dance classes are taught by dancers, yoga instructors are authorities on yoga, and so on. The equipment in these facilities is usually the best for your particular practice. In addition, the people taking classes with you share your avid interest in the practice. Who knows? Going to a class could be a great way to score a date, too. At least you know you and your date will have one thing in common.

In these types of studios, you can usually buy private sessions, semi-private sessions (with one or two other people), or group sessions. You may also be able to purchase single sessions or a package of sessions—the more you buy, the lower the price per class.

PERSONAL TRAINING FOCUS

The sole purpose of some gyms is to offer one-on-one personal training. These gyms have several trainers on staff and are sometimes owned by a group of trainers themselves. Each client is matched up with a trainer who best suits his or her needs. And if you don't know what your needs are, the staff can help steer you in the right direction. Training sessions are usually sold in packages of 10, 20, or more. Here again, the more sessions you buy, the lower your per-session rate.

THE LOWDOWN

THE CLUB MIX

A great way to keep your workout program fresh and fun is to mix it up by alternating visits to personal training gyms with sessions at class-focused studios.

GENDER SPECIFIC

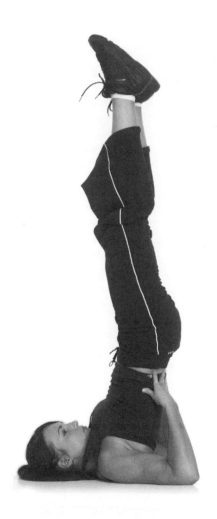

Some may feel uncomfortable working out with members of the opposite sex. To remedy that, there are a variety of gyms that cater specifically to men or women. One of the most popular examples of this, Curves, is based on an easy-to-use circuit training program. Curves is a fitness concept that is now available at over 9,000 locations around the world. It is a women-only program that promises results in a 30-minute workout, three times a week. Each Curves is independently owned but is meant to operate using the same model (kind of like a Starbucks for working out). The basic idea is to provide a comfortable place for women to work out and receive weight-loss guidance. There are no mirrors in the workout room, and the entire setup is made up of 8 to 13 machines arranged in a circular formation. Some locations offer nutritional counseling as well.

Curves does not offer any of the spa amenities other gyms include: no shower, no sauna, no child care. If you're a woman who'd like to get started on a road to fitness by following a guided program, and would enjoy working out in an environment with other women who have similar goals, the Curves program may be a great option for you.

MEMBERSHIPS AND CONTRACTS

Another way gyms differ is in the way they contractually operate. Most facilities offer a one-year or a two-year membership and give you the option to pay in full upon joining, or break the cost down into monthly installments—a longer commitment to the gym often means a lower monthly rate. Not included in your membership rate is usually some type of additional initiation fee. In most gyms, a contract is a commitment just like a lease on a rental apartment. You are basically tied to that gym for the amount of time you sign up for. There are ways of getting out of your contract, but trying to do so prematurely—that is, before the expiration date—will most likely cost you something.

THE LOWDOWN

THE COST OF A BREAKUP

Depending on what gym you belong to, getting out of your contract could mean different things. Some gyms simply ask that you give them advance notice of your departure and then let you go without charging hidden fees or asking too many questions. Others may require you to cover your dues for a month or two after your official last day. If you paid for a full year or more in advance, you will be refunded the balance from your last day once all penalty dues, if any, are covered. Some gyms may give you a hard time. They will make you prove to them that you are either injured or moving out of the area. You may be required to provide documents from doctors or bills with your new address in order for the gym to refund your money. Depending on the level of the gym's administrative organization, this process can take way too long and can become a big annoyance. The lesson: ask questions before signing anything, especially if you are thinking about relocating.

THE FEES

Another payment alternative that may be offered is the pay-as-you-go option, which involves a monthly fee but no contractual agreement as to how long you will remain a member. Don't think you automatically get out of paying an initiation fee by choosing this option. Facilities offering this type of membership usually require an initiation fee as well. And you can't

THE LOWDOWN

THE MONTH OFF

Just because you are not paying for your membership during your frozen month, don't be mistaken: your muscles and fat cells are not going to "freeze" along with it. Try not to stop working out completely. You should try to schedule maintenance workouts that are, perhaps, shorter than usual and that can be done behind your closed office door or in your home. Think in terms of remaining active. Remember, you are committing to a lifestyle of activity, not just to a membership at a gym. Several books are available that can give you simple ideas for working out outside of a gym. We've written one called *Body Bar: 133 Moves for Full-Body Fitness*

terminate your membership at any given moment either. You'll be required to give the gym notice (usually 30 days, but sometimes a shorter period) as a courtesy to let them know that you won't be returning the following month. The pay-as-you-go alternative is a great option if you're wary of commitment in general or unsure if the particular gym suits your personality and fitness goals. The danger with this type of membership is that by allowing an easy breach of contract, it facilitates breaking your commitment to getting in shape. Thirty days of paying for something you are not intending to use may not be on your list of taboos. Don't let this become your excuse for not sticking to your workout program.

THE FREEZE

What happens if your job requires you to be out of the country for the entire month of May and you don't want to pay for a gym membership you won't be using? Ask the staff at your gym about their membership freeze options. The amount of time you are allowed to extend that freeze varies from a minimum of 30 days to whatever time frame is agreed upon in the contract.

THE PACKAGE

What does a "membership" include? Again, the term varies greatly from facility to facility. The rate usually includes all or most classes. Sometimes the gym will offer a "specialty" program or classes taught by "celebrity" instructors, and these activities may command an additional fee.

Your membership will always enable you to use the strength training floor and all of its accoutrements, the cardio equipment, the locker room, the showers, and the like. (Keep in mind that you will usually need to bring your own lock, no matter what type of gym you join.) With the full-service, glamour gyms, your fee will include limitless use of fresh towels and a coat check for when you have extra baggage. Sometimes it will also include all the bottled water you need and laundry services, although these provisions are quite rare. With the full-service, basic gyms, you will sometimes need to pay a fee for the use of one of the gym's towels. At these places, you may need to pay for the coat check, and you can forget about getting laundry service.

In all gyms, hiring a personal trainer costs an additional fee, and the rate per session will depend on the level of experience of your trainer and how many sessions you purchase at a time. Most full-service gyms will offer you a free one-time fitness evaluation. Don't let this prospect scare

> ## THE LOWDOWN
> ### STRATEGIC TIMING
> A little secret about joining any facility is that you will tend to get more for your money if you join at the end of the month. Gyms are businesses, just like all others, and are usually trying to hit their new membership sales goals at the end of the month. This is the time when they are more likely to offer a number of extra perks to get you to join. For example, if a particular gym charges initiation fees on top of its rates, you may be able to get around them. The time of the year is also another tariff-determining factor. Many gyms drop their rates in January to be competitive during the New Year's resolution rush. If it's mid-December and you are looking to join a gym, wait a couple of weeks longer for a better rate. You may also be able to save in numbers. Try getting a friend to join with you or, better yet, try to get your company to work out a corporate rate with the gym (if one with another gym does not already exist). Joining at the corporate rate may save you tons of cash and help motivate your friends and coworkers to get in shape as well.

you. Having one done only means they will weigh you, take your blood pressure, measure your body fat, and perhaps test your strength, flexibility, and aerobic capacity. You will usually get a free one-hour training session upon joining as well. Child care, if available, is also usually free.

THE PERSONAL ROUTE

Hiring a personal trainer is a great option for many reasons. Personal trainers are like therapists. They are explicitly there for you; for the entire time they are on your clock. They are there to help you identify your specific goals, to help plan how to work toward those goals, and to motivate you. They are experts in their field and should be able to impart their experience and knowledge to help you. Sounds like quite an important job, no? It is. Shopping for a personal trainer who is right for you will require finding one with complementary training experiences and the proper education. More importantly, as with a therapist, you and your trainer must have a connection. You should feel completely comfortable sharing your fitness doubts, fears, and aspirations with this person. Furthermore, you should be able to readily bestow upon your trainer full confidence in his or her ability to lead you to your desired level of fitness.

THE COURSE OF ACTION

How you elect to structure your arrangement with a personal trainer is your call entirely. There are several options to consider. What course of action you choose to take basically depends on three things: your level of self-motivation, your ultimate goals for the sessions, and how much cash you're willing to dish out. Reflect on the following paradigms.

PARADIGM ONE: THE PERSONAL TRAINER

In this scenario, you will be surrendering the reins to your talented, trustworthy, and carefully selected trainer and pledging continual commitment to your work with her or him. In most situations, you meet with your trainer at least two to three times per week. He or she will guide you toward your initial goals while carefully plotting your progress and helping you to reevaluate and reassess your objectives as you move along. This is the most intensive, focused connection you could have with a trainer, and certainly it's the scenario that will reap the most rewards, should your financial hands be unbound. You will be making a full-on, timeless commitment to your training. You will be more likely to keep your appointments because skipping a training session will involve disappointing someone other than yourself (your trainer, your bank account). Whether you are highly motivated or questionably motivated, looking to refresh your current fitness routine or just getting started, you will not be disappointed with your choice.

Here's how this option stacks up in terms of your level of self-motivation, how much money you are willing to spend, and what you can expect to get out of the sessions. It's clear that you will need deep pockets to have a personal trainer in all three scenarios. But how you will use this trainer will depend on your level of motivation. For example, if you are questionably motivated, you'll need the trainer to be a "nudge," helping you to keep going to the sessions and pushing you to do the exercises correctly and get to the next level. If you're moderately motivated, you will want the trainer to guide you through the exercises every step of the way. However, if you're highly motivated, the trainer can serve to spot-check you, to see that you're doing the exercises correctly, and to fine-tune your workout.

SELF-MOTIVATION	Questionable	Moderate	High
POCKETS	Deep	Deep	Deep
SCENARIO	Need the constant guidance of trainer to stick to program	Just starting out and/or want constant guidance from trainer	Seeking company of trainer during sessions with added benefit of guidance

PARADIGM TWO: RENT-A-TRAINER

With this type of arrangement, you will retain the services of a personal trainer specializing in your desired area of focus for a set period of time. The longevity of your sessions would depend on your specific goal or goals and the sessions would end once those intended goals were achieved. We have highlighted a few specific examples below. In each case, success would be determined by your own ability to self-inspire and infuse the application of your new set of skills into your fitness practice. Your trainer will not be there to provide that extra dose of encouragement and make sure you keep pushing forward. This is an agreeable and very practical option for the moderately to highly self-motivated. Those lacking such heights of motivation risk the possibility of sweeping the rewards of their training under the rug and reverting to their old routine or simply calling it quits and resigning from working out completely. It also makes it possible for those with a limited budget to hire a personal trainer. This is a great and cost-effective way to keep your workouts fresh and stimulating, both physically and mentally. It is also a clever way to ensure you are executing exercises with proper technique and establishing a good baseline if working out is new to you.

SELF-MOTIVATION	Questionable	Moderate to high	Moderate to high	High
POCKETS	Doesn't matter. This is probably not the best option for you.	Shallow to deep	Shallow to deep	Shallow to deep
SCENARIO	N/A	Fitness enthusiast looking to learn how to do something new, like doing core work with cables, or searching for new ideas to avoid monotony	Looking to train for a specific event, such as a marathon	Novice needing help getting started

PARADIGM THREE:
THE TRAINER AS CONSULTANT

Imagine your personal trainer as a fitness consultant. In this situation, you would consult with your personal trainer every so often to evaluate your progress and revise your current program or introduce a new one. Your consultations could consist of one or more sessions. The amount of time in between your meetings would be determined by your specific needs. We have highlighted a few examples below. It would be up to you and your own self-inspiring abilities to infuse your new set of skills into your fitness practice, making this option an intelligent and penny-minding one for the moderately to highly self-motivated. Although your next meeting with your trainer would be a long one to four months away, the anticipation of the meeting would bestow upon you the motivation needed to master your new program and achieve your prescribed ambitions.

SELF-MOTIVATION	Questionable	Moderate to high	High
POCKETS	Doesn't matter. This is probably not the best option for you.	Shallow to deep	Shallow to deep
SCENARIO	N/A	Fitness enthusiast looking to take it to the next level or for fresh ideas for training	Novice needing help getting started

THE TRAINER INQUISITION

Ask, ask, and ask. What should you be asking? Here are some key questions that may help you find your match.

The inquisition should begin with the simplest question of all.

Why are you a personal trainer? Why do you do what you do?

Is the trainer passionate about his career or is personal training just a side job until he gets a big break as an actor in a major motion picture? This latter scenario does not necessarily mean that this trainer will be derelict in his duties, but it does indicate that perhaps the trainer's focus lies elsewhere.

What are your qualifications?

Your potential trainer should be educated in her field and be able to walk the talk. Find out what your trainer's personal experiences for training have been. What does she do for herself? You want someone who has had personal experience with training and is reaping the benefits of its positive results. You want a trainer who inspires and motivates you through her own experiences and actions.

How long have you been in this business?

If your trainer is just starting out, that does not mean that he won't end up being a phenomenal motivator and trainer. What it does indicate is that you may be an experimental subject— a "guinea pig"—for this person, especially if you have very particular needs. If you are pregnant, selecting a novice to the training field to train you might not be the best move; he might not have the right experiences to work with you. If you do have a special need, ask the trainer if he has experience with your particular need. And if you are looking to train for a specific event, like running a marathon, look for a trainer with experience with that sport. If the trainer you are interviewing doesn't run, perhaps you should continue your search.

Ask around. Personal testimonies are probably the best, most authentic indicators of quality. Talk to your potential trainer's other clients. Get a feel for how long they have been training with this person, what type of training they do, how happy they are, and if they have been moving toward their desired results.

THE INSIDE SCOOP

Become a private detective. Keep an eye on trainers of interest while they are in action with clients. Do they pay attention to what the clients are doing throughout the session, or are the trainers looking around the room for friends or prospective dates? Do the clients look content with their workouts? Are the trainers more interested in carrying on a conversation and gossiping about last night's affairs or taking cell phone calls than in making sure their clients are performing each exercise with precision? On another note, discretion while spying is advised. Avoid distracting the trainers and trainees or being the cause of a possible accident.

When investing in training sessions, don't buy too many sessions right off the bat. Get firsthand experience first. In the end, what may work for someone else may not work for you. Start with five sessions to see how you feel and how you vibe with your trainer. Some gyms will allow you to use your purchased sessions with any trainer in the gym.

Clear communication is fundamental. Make an effort to clearly express to your trainer what you aim to accomplish through your sessions. Doing so will help your trainer counsel you in the direction of your ambitions and compose a fitting personalized program that will meet your needs. For example, if your goals include becoming stronger and decreasing body fat, your program will include a combination of resistance training and cardiovascular conditioning. If your goal is to be able to run a marathon, however, your program will call for a different balance of resistance training and cardiovascular conditioning, all of which will be directly related to running.

We'll help you delineate a set of goals in Chapter 2.

GOALS:
THE NUTS
AND BOLTS

2

What we can or cannot do, what we consider possible or impossible, is rarely a function of our true capacity. It is more like a function of our beliefs about who we are.

TONY ROBBINS

SO, you've decided to join a gym. Why? Whether you realize it or not, the reason is that you want to change something about yourself. What is your fitness destiny?

THE POINT

It's easier to save money if you know you're saving for something of great desire, like a new flat-screen TV or a tropical beach vacation. Goals help motivate us. They keep us connected to the end result. Goals are the reason reality TV shows, which subject people to extremely uncomfortable situations, exist. Why else would people allow themselves to be televised while eating bugs, if not for the jackpot at the end? Create a vivid picture of your goals and develop a strong emotional attachment to them. It is these emotional attachments that will invigorate your forward-moving crusades.

Goals foster efficient and focused action. If you're in New York and your goal is to drive to Florida, you wouldn't need to map out rest areas in Colorado. In the same way, if your fitness goal is to gain muscle mass, you need to follow a muscle-building map to achieve that goal and you would want to spend more time lifting weights than pedaling on a stationary bike.

MENTAL MUSCLE

How ludicrous it seems to think that people put so much time and effort into the upkeep of their cars, homes, and wardrobes, when their most prized possessions—their bodies—are neglected.

THE RECIPE FOR SUCCESS

Unlike plotting out a road trip, identifying the kinds of changes you would like to make through working out and figuring out how to achieve those goals may be a bit ambiguous. Here's a way to think about your goals and how to work toward reaching them.

THE KEY INGREDIENTS

THE ULTIMATE ASPIRATION

This is your fantasy goal. It is something specific you want for yourself that is so huge, you are almost afraid to say it out loud or to admit it to anyone besides yourself. For example, winning the Tour de France, looking like Han Solo instead of Jabba the Hut, or not being unanimously elected to play Santa Claus at your kid's holiday show for the fifth year in a row. To determine your ultimate aspiration, ask yourself, if you were the epitome of fitness, what would you be like? What types of activities would you participate in? Would you play your favorite sport,

maybe join your local basketball team? Perhaps it's about being fit enough to be able to keep up with your kids. What would you feel like? What would your clothes fit like? Can you see this image of yourself in your mind's eye? Hold on to this visual and take note of even the smallest details.

THE LOWDOWN

MENTAL POWER

The Cleveland Clinic Foundation did a study on mental workouts and found that patients who simply imagined they were flexing their muscles for 12 weeks, five times a week, had a 13.5 percent increase in muscle strength. These results lasted three months after stopping the mental training. The point is, set your mind to what you are doing. Focus. It will help bring you the results you desire.

THE MIDPOINTS ARE YOUR MARKERS

Midpoints are measurable checkpoints that ensure you are on the right track, heading toward your ultimate aspiration. Reaching a checkpoint is like a mini-victory that will help boost your confidence, motivate you onward, and help you to begin seeing yourself differently. For example, if you are driving on an unfamiliar road en route to a new destination, you look for signs to make sure you're going in the right direction. Once you begin to see these signs, you feel reassured that you're nearing the desired destination and you grow increasingly excited as you anticipate reaching your target. Midpoints make the ultimate aspiration feel like a possible reality. If your ultimate aspiration is to lose 100 pounds, perhaps your first-month midpoint goal would be to lose five pounds. Five pounds down and you are on your way. Remember to reward yourself. This is super-important. When defining the midpoints, also plan out the rewards you will give yourself once you reach them. The rewards can be anything you would really look forward to, like a new pair of shoes or a massage with your favorite therapist. They should make you feel proud and excited about moving forward, and not be detrimental to your ultimate goal. Try not to rekindle bad eating habits or sedentary behaviors.

THE BASIC ELEMENTS

These are your specific daily actions, your directions. What are you going to do to get to where you want to go? Let's get back to the Tour de France example: If winning is your ultimate aspiration, purchasing a bike and learning to ride it would be a couple of your first basic elements. The basic elements include all the things you need to do to reach your midpoints and then your ultimate aspiration. They also include all the things you need to stop doing (like not eating donuts for breakfast or not driving to a destination that is within walking distance).

A GOAL-SETTING EXAMPLE

THE ULTIMATE ASPIRATION

I have marked my calendar. It is January 1. My next New Year's Eve, I will decrease my body fat percentage from 35 to 15 percent. I want to be able to see, without the help of sheer imagination, my six-pack, and be able to keep up with my kids. I will increase my overall strength and self-confidence.

THE MIDPOINTS

By April 1, I will have decreased my body fat to 50 percent at most. From today through April 1, I will go to the gym two to three days a week. My reward for achieving these midpoint goals will be a new pair of shoes.

By July 1, my body fat will be 25 percent at most. From April 2 through July 1, I will go to the gym three to four days a week. My reward for achieving these midpoint goals will be tickets to a show.

By October 1, my body fat will be 20 percent at most. From July 2 through October 1, I will go to the gym four to five days a week. My reward for achieving these midpoint goals will be treating myself to a massage at my favorite spa.

By December 31, my body fat will be 15 percent or lower (yeah!). From October 2 through December 31, I will go to the gym five to six days a week. My reward for achieving these midpoint goals will be a week on the beach in Hawaii.

THE BASIC ELEMENTS

I will hire a trainer.

Every Sunday I will evaluate my previous week's happenings, progress, and disappointments. I will write in my planner the specific time of my workouts for each day. For each day, I will write exactly what I will do in each of these workouts.

(For example, Monday—Take Gregg Cook's Urban Rebounding class at 7 a.m. Wednesday—Meet with my trainer. Friday—Same as Monday's.)

I will cut all fried foods from my diet.

I will make sure I include fresh veggies in my lunch and dinner meals.

THE INSIDE SCOOP

BE SPECIFIC

Make every goal you set as specific as possible, and include actual numbers as guidelines. For example, determine the exact amount of body fat percentage you want to lose. Know that you would like to run an 8-minute mile instead of a 10-minute mile.

BE AMBITIOUS

Set challenging goals for yourself. Don't stand in your own way of becoming the best you can be by setting goals that are too easily attainable. At the same time, make sure your goals are attainable. Talk to a personal trainer who can help you evaluate what is possible in a realistic time frame and perhaps guide you along in this process.

BE FLEXIBLE

As you move forward in your workout program, be sure to continually reevaluate the goals you set out to attain. A good time to do so is when you reach one of your midpoints. The edges surrounding your goals should be malleable. Your goals will morph from one thing to another as you change and progress both physically and mentally. What you thought were your physical and mental limits with working out might end up being merely the tip of the iceberg. Let's say, for example, you join a gym and start with the strict goal of making it to the gym for one hour, two times a week. You may find that you thoroughly enjoy going to the gym five days a week but prefer to limit your time every other day to 30 minutes. The pervasive and long-familiar goal of "losing weight" may have been your initial goal, but after falling in love with that kick-butt spin class, you may strive to train for a race and shift your focus in that direction.

BE A VISIONARY

Your mind is more powerful than you can possibly imagine. In your mind's eye, see yourself as if you were already exactly as you would like to be. The only way you'll ever get there is if you get out of your own way and believe in yourself. This truism is of utmost importance. If you limit the mental image you have of yourself, you also limit what you may become.

GOALS: THE NUTS AND BOLTS

HAVE A PLAN

Before you go to the gym, create a workout program for the day. Plan out precisely what you want to do. Doing so will make the time spent at the gym much more efficient and productive. It will structure your workouts in general and help you reach your goals more quickly. For example, figure out how much time you are allotting to working out. Next, identify what type of training you are going to concentrate on. Will it be cardiovascular training, or will you be working on resistance training? Even more specific, if dedicating your workout solely to cardiovascular training, is it going to be a day of endurance work or intervals? If you plan to devote yourself to resistance training for the day, delineate whether your lower body, upper body, or full body will be the focus. Know your planned workout thoroughly: determine exactly what exercises you'll be doing, exactly what weights you'll use, how many reps you'll do, and how much rest you'll allow in between sets.

BE ORGANIZED

Set aside a time every Sunday evening to evaluate your past workout week and determine your basic elements for the following week. Reflecting on the prior week will give you some insight into how to design your workout in future weeks. Again, be very specific. All of the time you spend at the gym should be accounted for. Invest in a fitness journal. Writing out your workout plans will make them feel like more of a reality. It will attach a sense of importance to what you are doing and give reference points to look back on. On top of that, detailed daily workout plans are definitely more concrete and easier to follow than those simply committed to memory.

PIECES OF THE GYM PUZZLE

3

THERE ARE four distinct facets of a gym, each with very different characteristics and functions:

1   RESISTANCE TRAINING

2   CARDIOVASCULAR TRAINING

3   CORE STRENGTH, BALANCE AND STABILITY

4   FLEXIBILITY AND STRETCHING

THE LOWDOWN

THE BALANCING ACT

Life is all about creating balance. What is a see without a saw? Who is Ben without Jerry or Abbott without Costello? Your body, mind, and spirit all work in concert. Your existence and experience of life is a choreographed masterpiece of the three. It follows that the way in which you train your body should also be balanced. This balance is precisely what it means to be truly healthy—to be strong, flexible, nimble, quick, smooth, and graceful. It is equally important to dedicate time to all types of training: cardiovascular, core, strength, balance and stability, and flexibility and stretching.

RESISTANCE TRAINING

The importance of adding resistance training to a workout repertoire is becoming increasingly acknowledged. (This goes for women as well as men.) So what, exactly, does resistance training mean? The concept is fairly simple: resistance training is the disciplined addition of weight, or "resistance," to exercises in order to train your muscles to have the capacity to handle more; in other words, you will be training them to become stronger. As with anything else, the more you do something, the better you get at it, and the less of a challenge

it becomes. As you practice, your body adapts to the weights or resistance, and you, in turn, are able to handle more.

THE KICKBACKS

- Stronger muscles
- Stronger bones (and reduced risk of developing osteoporosis)
- Stable joints (avoid orthopedic problems)
- Decreased chance of injury
- Increased resting metabolic rate (burn more calories while doing nothing: your body will be a fat-burning furnace)
- Reduced risk of diabetes
- Leaner and sculpted body (the potential "drawback" is developing a mirror obsession)
- Increased energy
- Perform daily tasks and chores with greater ease
- Increased self-confidence
- Increased ability in sports

TRUTH BE TOLD

Misconceptions about pumping iron run amok in the world of the sedentary—even some of the most active individuals are quite misinformed. These misconceptions have earned a broad-based following, even among those who lead lifestyles packed with cardiovascular activities, and provide the seemingly perfect excuses for not lifting weights. As your personal fitness crusaders, we're here to liberate you from such fallacies. Strength training is a vital part of becoming fit and is also essential to maintaining your hard-earned fitness results. Among other things, by practicing resistance training, you're teaching your

muscles and your brain how to move with increased strength, fluidity, and safety in your day-to-day life. So, without further ado, let's examine some of the most common myths about strength training—and put them to rest, once and for all.

MYTH: If I do a million crunches, I will develop a super six-pack and lose inches around my waistline.

TRUTH

The good news is that this concept is true; you will develop your six-pack. The bad news is that you'll need to do more than crunches in order to unveil it. Your abdominal muscles are already there. Unfortunately, no one will ever know it unless you melt away the fat covering them up. There is no such thing as spot reducing. This goes for any of the "trouble spots" you are trying to work on—jiggly upper arms, inner thighs that rub against each other, doughy back fat, and so on ... you get the idea. You can't tell your body exactly where to burn fat. The basic idea is to melt away fat all around by burning more calories than you take in through a combination of resistance training, cardiovascular exercise, and smart eating.

MYTH: *If I train, I will get big and bulky.*

TRUTH

Maybe and maybe not. There are different types of training geared toward attaining specific results. If you're a woman, chances are you won't bulk up because your body does not produce enough testosterone for your muscles to grow that big. So, unless you decide to unnaturally and illegally juice it up, you don't have to worry about unwanted bulk. Another factor to take into consideration is your genetic makeup. If you have a naturally stick-thin, sinewy frame reminiscent of classic beanpoles such as Olive Oyl, you'll get stronger and see muscle build for sure, but you won't develop the bulging muscles of those born with a more Popeye-style body type. On the other hand, if you naturally have a muscular build, you'll always have that muscular build. You can shape your body in the sense that you can become leaner and stronger, but your body type will not change. For example, if you have short legs and a long torso, you'll never be able to alter those proportions. Love and respect the body you have and make it the best it can be by being active and maintaining a well-rounded fitness practice.

MYTH: *Doing cardio work will take the place of resistance training.*

TRUTH

They are not the same. Cardio work focuses principally on the heart, as the name implies. It conditions your heart to become stronger and work more efficiently. Resistance training focuses on building lean muscles so that you can move with more strength and protect your joints. Both types of exercise will burn calories. The increased calorie-burning effect of a typical cardio session essentially ends at the end of a workout. (This does not include very high intensity anaerobic interval training.) After a thorough resistance training session, your body will continue to burn calories at an increased rate for hours. Both types of exercises are absolutely necessary and work synergistically.

PIECES OF THE GYM PUZZLE

MYTH: If I stop training, my muscles will turn to fat.

Muscle fibers and fat cells are like apples and oranges, completely different. If you stop exercising and continue to eat the same way you did when you were exercising, all those calories you will no longer be burning as fuel for energy will be stored as fat. At the same time, if you do not use your muscles, they will shrink. Your muscles don't turn into fat. They just shrink and become cloaked with fat.

TRUTH

MYTH: Squats and lunges will hurt my knees.

Think exactly the opposite. You need strong muscles surrounding your joints in order to support them. Strong quadriceps and hamstrings will support your knees, and squats and lunges, done correctly, are essential in strengthening them.

TRUTH

MYTH: I can't do any resistance training. I don't want to build my muscle. I am a dancer and need to be flexible.

Flexibility training should be balanced with resistance training. A strong muscle acts as a bodyguard for the joints and will decrease the probability of overstretching and associated injuries.

TRUTH

THE INSIDE SCOOP

- Warm up. Warming up is the process of raising your body temperature and getting the muscles ready to work out. Warm muscles contract with more force and relax with less effort. In other words, in your workout, muscles that have been sufficiently warmed up will be stronger and less tense. The idea is to get blood flowing freely through the muscles. Blood provides the oxygen and fuel necessary for muscles to work properly. Warming up will increase the elasticity of your muscles and lubricate your joints. You'll be more flexible and better able to avoid injury. The warm-up process is also a great opportunity to clear your mind and bring your focus to the work you are about to do. Simple examples of a good warm-up include a brisk walk or a leisurely bike ride (perhaps en route to the gym). Engaging in movements similar to what you plan to do during your session, but at a lower intensity, is also a clever idea. We personally like warming up with 10- to 15-minute core-centered workouts.

- Machines are a dependable way to get started with resistance training. Because all of their parts are fused together in one spaceship-like contraption, machines eliminate the danger of dropping loose parts on your toes (or someone else's). Dropping is a hazard that exists when using free weights. Machines provide a preset and specific range of motion and will safely guide your movements. Get acquainted with the machines first, to get used to the mechanics of each movement. Incorporate the use of dumbbells, bars, and the like, once you're comfortable with the proper way to execute the exercises on the machines. Dumbbells and bars are slightly more advanced, because in using them you are also practicing balance, coordination, and joint stabilization. Start out with no weight or lighter weights when first practicing a move. To get the optimum results, your form *must* be flawless and you need to be able to get a full range of motion from each exercise. Throwing caution to the wind and beginning in another way is foolish. Don't be shy about not looking as strong as the person beside you or appearing a bit odd when practicing a movement with no weights. Remember, your workout, unlike so many other things we do in life, is all about you. Besides, there are so many bizarre-looking things going on in a gym at any given moment that surely no one

THE LOWDOWN

DRESS REHEARSAL

Think of your everyday life when training. Imagine you are going on a quick weekend island getaway and are lifting your carry-on bag into the overhead compartment of the airplane. Essentially, you are doing a squat with a bicep curl and a shoulder press. Exercises that target more than one muscle group at a time are the most efficient and functional.

PIECES OF THE GYM PUZZLE

THE LOWDOWN

ENDURE

As a newcomer to strength training, it's a good idea to begin your program with a focus on muscle endurance. Use light, manageable weights and perform a high number of repetitions (approximately 12 to 15 reps). As you become comfortable with this, shift your focus to muscle strength—increase the amount of weight you're using and lower the number of repetitions (approximately 8 to 12 reps).

will notice the seeming peculiarities of your actions.

- When working more than one muscle group in a session, we suggest starting from the largest muscle group and working your way down to the smallest. The larger muscles will consume the most energy, and putting them to work while they are fresh will allow you to get the most out of them. Here is the breakdown—lower body, back/chest, shoulders, triceps, and biceps. The smaller muscles will help support you while working the larger ones. If you've already tired out the little guys, you won't be able to work the big guys as efficiently when it's their turn.

- If you're doing multiple exercises for one muscle group, start with the exercises that are most challenging for you. You will have more strength and mental focus to complete them. Finish with the exercises about which you are most confident.

- Maintain control throughout the entire movement of the exercise. Pay extra attention to lowering the weight—this motion is just as important as the lifting. Our bodies need to develop strength when lowering weight in the direction of gravity. Think of lifting and lowering a heavy box. If you don't have the strength to control lowering

that box, opportunities for accidents present themselves.

- Always take time to cool down so your body has a chance to remove by-products of working out that may leave your muscles feeling an achy stiffness and soreness the next day.

- Stretching is a big component of cooling down and is an essential part of a balanced training program. It encourages a full range of motion in the joints and leaves you feeling blissfully relaxed.

- Stretching a warm muscle is much more effective and safer than stretching a cold one. Steer away from stretching cold muscles. If you're doing nothing but stretching for the day, warm up for 5 to 10 minutes first. Think of your muscles as Silly Putty. Silly Putty stretches with much more freedom and ease when it is warm. Think of your muscles in the same way.

CARDIOVASCULAR TRAINING

Cardiovascular training is to the heart what resistance training is to the other muscles of your body. It increases the demands on the heart in order to strengthen it and help it to work more efficiently. Here is a very rough idea of how it all works. The heart is in partnership with the lungs. If you image your cardiovascular system as a transport system, blood is the vehicle that distributes all of the energy-creating resources (oxygen, carbohydrates, and fats) throughout the body and the heart is the central source of power for this vehicle. The lungs are the recycling center, where the blood drops off wastes (carbon dioxide and water) and picks up fresh resources (oxygen). The veins, arteries, and capillaries are the passageways that connect all the components of the cardiovascular system to the working muscles.

THE KICKBACKS

- Increased VO2 max (your body's ability to utilize oxygen for energy)
- More efficient heart (your heart will pump a higher volume of blood with fewer beats)
- Slows your resting heart rate
- Decreased risk of coronary heart disease (a powerful pump of blood through the arteries helps keep them open and clear)
- Lowering levels of bad cholesterol (LDL)
- Raising levels of good cholesterol (HDL)
- Increased recovery rate (helps your body bounce back faster after strenuous activities)
- Leaner body
- Increased energy
- Perform daily tasks/chores with added ease
- Increased self-confidence
- Increased ability in sports
- Mood lifter (reduces anxiety and depression)

TRUTH BE TOLD

Now it's time to tackle some common myths about cardiovascular training.

MYTH: I don't do cardio because I want to build muscle.

As a beginner, your body uses mostly carbohydrates and a little fat as a main source of fuel during cardiovascular activities. Very little muscle is broken down to be used as energy. If your focus is on building strength, most of your time should be spent on strength training, but cardiovascular activities are still important.

TRUTH

MYTH: I shouldn't eat anything after cardiovascular exercise because it will undo some of the great calorie-burning effects of the workout.

Your total caloric intake throughout the day will essentially be the same whether you eat right after the workout or three hours later. You may actually be better off eating or drinking something high in carbs right after a cardio workout. Immediately following a workout, your body will use what you consume to replenish muscle fuel stores much more efficiently than an hour or more after. Examples of good muscle fuel replenishers are a small banana or a bowl of oatmeal, or a sports drink such as Amino Vital. (Check out their Web site, www.amino-vital.com.)

TRUTH

MYTH: *Cardiovascular exercise is the fastest way to lose weight.*

TRUTH

A combination of cardiovascular and resistance training is the most efficient and fastest way to lose weight. If there was a magic formula, in our opinion, this would be it (plus a dosage of core work and flexibility training, of course). They work collaboratively.

MYTH: *I need to work in the "fat-burning zone" in order to burn fat and lose weight.*

TRUTH

The fact is that at lower intensities—that is, the "fat-burning zone"—your body uses fat as a predominant source of fuel. As you increase intensity, your body begins to use carbohydrates more predominantly but also burns more calories overall. The higher the intensity of your workout, the more calories you burn, and this includes fat. If you do the math, at higher intensities you would be burning just about the same amount of fat, but many more calories overall, and this is the main point. Any extra, unused calories are basically stored in your body as fat. So, if you are looking to burn fat, don't be afraid to work hard.

MYTH: *More sweat equals more calories burned and a better workout.*

TRUTH

Not so. If this were true, anyone living in hot climates would automatically be in great shape. When your body overheats, it is not able to work as efficiently. Basically, you want the warmth in your body during a workout to be generated from your workout, not from external conditions. You may feel like you are working extra hard because of the discomfort of the heat and the sweat dripping off you, but it is just that, discomfort. Sweating is fine, but is certainly not the best way to rate the value of a particular workout.

THE INSIDE SCOOP

• Just as with resistance training, before getting into your cardio workout, warm up for 5 to 10 minutes. See "Resistance Training: The Inside Scoop" for the reasons why.

THE LOWDOWN

PERSPIRING NOTES

Have you ever wondered why your pores seem to leak when you are hot? Perspiring is your body's natural cooling system. Perspiration is made up of water, as well as minerals called electrolytes—sodium, potassium, magnesium, to name a few—that help keep the fluids of the body in a balanced state. When you sweat for extended periods of time (over an hour), rehydration is critical. So, drink plenty of water and consume sports drinks to replenish lost electrolytes. Our favorite, Amino Vital (see www.amino-vital.com), will also give you the added benefits of amino acids (the building blocks of protein), which will help combat muscle fatigue, and expedite the recovery and rebuilding process.

• Explore. Try different endurance activties, such as running, cycling, or rowing, to find the ones that really delight you. You never really know which activity you'll enjoy until you give it a go. Who knows? You may discover that you're a late-blooming marathon runner or cyclist at heart.

• At the start of a cardiovascular training program, err on the side of easy to moderate workouts lasting 20 to 30 minutes long, plus a warm-up and cool-down. If your schedule permits and objectives coincide, work your way up toward longer and more intense workouts. Remember, marathon runners who seem as if they could gracefully go on forever did not start out being able to run as long as they do. They ran shorter distances in order to work up to it.

HEART RATE MONITORS AND ZONE TRAINING

There are two parts to a heart rate monitor, the strap and the watch. The rubber strap that is worn around the chest (almost like a bra strap without the cups) is what picks up your heartbeat. The watch worn around the wrist (like any other watch) documents the signals sent from the strap and interprets the data according to various pieces of personal information (such as age, activity level, and gender).

Many heart rate monitors are able to lead you through some simple physical tests in order to determine your zones—ranges of heart rates that correspond to different levels of intensity during workouts. There are benefits to working within each of the zones. One is not better than another, and all are important for specific reasons. Learn to associate the sensations you feel within a zone to be able to identify and manipulate the intensity of your workouts. Here's a rundown of the zones:

Zone 1—the Leisure Zone. This is the starting point. In this zone, your workout will feel easy, fun, and relaxing. Breathing is effortless. Working within this zone will lower blood pressure, help with weight loss, and aid in stress management. The calorie-burn rate at this level, however, is relatively low and working strictly at this level will not improve your performance.

Zone 2—the Moderate Zone. In this zone, your workout will feel comfortable and your breathing is easy. You may notice a little bit of moisture developing on your brow. In addition to the benefits of working in zone 1, zone 2 activities increase the amount of blood, oxygen, and nutrients delivered to the muscles, fortifying the heart and lungs.

Zone 3—the Aerobic Zone. You'll know when you've entered this zone when you start to really sweat and your breathing becomes noticeably heavier. You're "comfortably uncomfortable" and the workout feels tough but sustainable. Working in zone 3 capitalizes on all of the benefits of zones 1 and 2 and in addition will increase the volume of oxygen consumed, and overall muscle endurance.

PIECES OF THE GYM PUZZLE

Zone 4—the Threshold Zone. This feels very tough, and breathing is difficult. You are training at a high intensity. Even the most conditioned athletes have trouble keeping this up for extended periods of time. Training in this zone will give you the added benefit of increasing your muscles' tolerance to lactic acid.

Zone 5—the Red Zone. This is an extremely high-intensity zone and is not recommended for beginners. Training in this zone is important for maximizing speed and strength, but is taxing and may cause damage to your body if done with poor form.

Talk to someone trained in this subject matter to learn more about zones and training and be careful not to become a slave to the numbers displayed by your heart rate monitor. Your heart rate will be affected by many different variables on any given day. The monitor does not personally know you and will not be able to factor in these outside elements. In addition to using a heart rate monitor to gauge your level of exertion, there are a few other vitals signs you'll want to keep tabs on as you explore activities in the various zones.

Breath rate—The body is really such an intelligent creation. It is able to relay a wealth of information to you if you just pay it a bit of attention. Your breath rate is one of the most honest, objective, and reliable feedback mechanisms for gauging exercise intensity. You should make it a habit to note your breath rate whether you are using a heart rate monitor or not. Most training should be done at the Aerobic Zone; an intensity where breathing is noticeably increased, but controllable. Your experience should range from being able to talk comfortably on the easier side, to being uncomfortable to talk on the harder side. At higher heart rate zones, such as the Threshold Zone, your breathing is labored And you'd most likely choose to avoid talking if at all possible. In the Red Zone, you are breathing uncontrollably, "sucking wind."

Rate of perceived exertion (RPE)—This self-assessment scale, developed by Gunner Borg, allows you to identify how hard you feel you are working. Essentially, the scale associates a range of sensations (body heat, breath rate, and overall extent of discomfort) with numbers in order to help identify levels of intensity. The scale begins at level 6, "no exertion at all," and ends at 20, "maximal exertion." In our workouts, we simplify this scale to a range of 1 to 10, 1 reflecting "no exertion" and 10 reflecting "maximal exertion."

All in all, as your fitness program leads you through the different zones, it's a good idea to use a combination of the methods described above to gauge the intensity of your efforts. Try them all and find the combo that works best for you.

- Consider purchasing a heart rate monitor. It is a great feedback mechanism and a great way to help keep you focused throughout your workout. It shows you how your heart is being affected by the activity in which you are engaging. Over time, it will also help you keep track of your progress and paint a clear picture of the positive conditioning effects on your cardiovascular system.

- If you have knee, back, or hip issues, try lower-impact activities such as riding a stationary bike or an indoor cycling class, swimming, the elliptical machine, or an urban rebounding class.

- Pay attention to the innate intelligence of your body. If something feels very wrong, it probably is. If you feel nauseous or light-headed during your workout, listen to your body—and back off, or seriously consider ending that activity for the day. Also, remember that muscle soreness is not equivalent to a "bad" pain.

Examples of potentially dangerous sensations you shouldn't ignore during your workout:

- **Dizziness**
- **Light-headedness**
- **Sharp pain**
- **Seeing birds or stars**
- **Fainting (of course)**
- **Nausea**

Examples of positive sensations (however uncomfortable):

- **Muscle burning (may seem close to intolerable at times—this is fine)**
- **Controllable heavy breathing (please refrain from recreating inappropriate sounds in the gym— you know what we're talking about . . . more on offensive sounds in Chapter 6).**
- **A strong desire to give up**

KEEPING IT FRESH

Repetition can make you feel crazy. Doing the same thing over and over again can make any activity—even the ones you were once giddy about—feel cumbersome. Physical activities can have the same effect. Much like the law of diminishing returns, the positive mental and physical effects of repetitive activity begin to diminish. Avoid the monotony by simply trying different activities and thinking of your workout in different ways. Here are some ways you can mix things up:

The most obvious is to sample different activities or classes regularly.

THE LOWDOWN

CONSCIOUSNESS

An awakened state of attention will foster the best results at the gym (or anything you do, for that matter). Approach your workout with a ready, willing, and able mind-set.

If you want to do a 30-minute cardio workout on the machines and tend to get bored doing the same thing for the duration of your workout, try this: Do 10 minutes on a treadmill, 10 minutes on a stationary bike, and 10 minutes on the elliptical machine. It will make the time fly by and keep your body guessing.

Keep your workouts invigorating by using inspirational mantras. Before arriving at the gym, write out three to five positive affirmations. They could be anything that excites or exhilarates you. Some examples are "I can do it," "I am strong," "I am in perfect health," or "I will succeed." Try repeating each mantra to yourself for a minute or two at a time. Go through each of your affirmations for the duration of your workout. You may find that some are more motivating than others. If so, try infusing the greater motivators into your mix of mantras for longer periods of time.

Listening to music that motivates and drives you while working out helps to motivate you and keep you driven. It sounds foolish ... we know ... but sometimes this means stepping out of your musical box, extending your musical antennas, and trying out different genres of music—sample some tunes that are completely unlike what you normally listen to while lounging around sipping a glass of wine. Try playing games with your music during your workout by doing something different for each song. For example, if you are on a stationary bike, crank up the resistance while maintaining the same pedal speed for every other song.

Add extensive or intensive intervals to your cardio training once or twice a week. How?

EXTENSIVE INTERVALS: Do a series of long (3 to 10 minutes), intense intervals that are immediately followed by moderate periods lasting the same amount of time. For example, if you are running on the treadmill, speed up to a pace you would have a difficult time maintaining for more than the time allotted. Slow back down to a moderate pace for the same amount of time.

INTENSIVE INTERVALS: *This is an advanced form of training, and is not recommended for novices.* Do a series of short (30- to 90-second), very high intensity intervals that are immediately followed by rest periods lasting twice that amount of time. For example, if you are running on the treadmill, speed up to a sprint like pace that you would have an extremely hard time maintaining for more than the time allotted and would leave you breathless. Slow back down to a comfortable pace for twice that time.

THE NOTRE DAME

Think of your body as an extraordinary piece of architecture——say, one of the amazing cathedrals of Europe. The amount of time it took to build many of these cathedrals often exceeded a hundred years. Throughout these years, the builders patiently held on to and followed the ultimate plan to erect the structure as envisioned. Many of these cathedrals, built hundreds of years ago, are standing strongly to this day. The architecture and aesthetic of each one is unique and remarkable. To achieve such longevity, it is imperative that the foundation be solid. Crucial, too, is the need for all sides of the building to be equally strong. When we work out, we should think of ourselves as "body architects." To properly develop a solid fitness foundation takes patience and dedication. You are building the groundwork upon which all of your future fitness endeavors will grow. Careful attentiveness to practicing a well-rounded fitness program will build strength, grace, and magnificence from all perspectives.

CORE STRENGTH

It is time to get back to basics. We've bicep curled, triceps dipped, and calf raised our way around what working out is really about. Sure, carefully sculpted limbs are easy on the eyes, are fun to touch, and will help you lift and lower, or push and pull. The question is, what can they do for you if you lack a strong base or core? When the sun is setting on your years of youth, it is your core that will keep you standing tall. Core training has become an important trend in the fitness world. While there are many fitness fads that come and go more quickly than the beat of an allegro composition, this one is here to stay. And the reason why core training will remain at the heart of a well-balanced fitness plan is simple and sensible: the core is the center, the foundation, from which everything else stems. It is made up of all of your abdominal muscles and the back muscles that help mobilize and stabilize the spine and connect to the shoulder and hip joints. It is what holds you upright and steady, and it supports and enhances all of your movements.

Core training is the strengthening and conditioning of those muscles as both movers and stabilizers. Both functions are equally important. Strong core muscles as movers will help rotate, flex, and extend the spine, and will connect movement throughout the body. Strong core muscles as stabilizers provide a power-generating foundation for movement and will support good posture for a pain-free back.

THE KICKBACKS

- **Healthier back**
- **Better posture**
- **Decreased chance of injuries (particularly back injuries)**
- **Improved performance (power, technique, and coordination) in *all* activities (for example, pedal stroke on a bike, tennis swings, karate kicking, and lifting increasingly heavier weights)**

TRUTH BE TOLD

While everyone is interested in a sexy, flat stomach, the most common advice on how to achieve one isn't always accurate. Let's examine some myths about these core exercises and set the record straight.

MYTH: Crunches are the pillar of all core exercises and will result in the ever-so-sexy six-pack.

TRUTH

Crunches isolate the rectus abominus (the six-pack) while neglecting other core muscles that are equally important. The truth is that we should consider all of the core muscles as one muscle group working together, as opposed to muscles working separately. We should, in turn, train them as such. Standing core work (such as exercises done with cables) in general is more functional than floor-based core exercises. It engages all core muscles in a way that mimics how they will be used in your daily life. Ask a trainer to show you a few moves. Planks are also great (see "Planks" in Chapter 6).

MYTH: I do core work because I want to lose fat around my waistline.

TRUTH

There is no such thing as spot reduction. We don't mean to sound like a broken record, but this misconception is so deeply entrenched, we feel further clarification is in order. Core work is a phenomenal way to strengthen your abdominals and back muscles, but doing these exercises alone will not serve to "reduce" you in size. Only the combination of a well-balanced training program and smart eating habits will help you trim down all around.

THE INSIDE SCOOP

- Make regular core training a habit. It should be a priority, not an afterthought.

- Schedule your core work at the beginning of your training session while you're still wholeheartedly focused and enthusiastic about the physical challenges to follow. A little core training is a brilliant thing to do as a warm-up. For example, make front and side planks and a bridge your signature moves at the beginning of every training session.

- Keep your core muscles intrigued and ever-stimulated. Add inventive elements to your core training by learning to incorporate fun tools like cables, the Physio Ball, medicine balls, and the BOSU into your curriculum. (For more on this equipment, see Chapter 5.)

- We all know how precious time is. Don't waste it. Make the most of the time you have by sneaking core moves in between exercises that train other muscle groups.

- Be kind to your core muscles. After an intense core training session, treat them as you would all your other muscle groups: give them a day of rest and allow them to recover before the next workout.

TRIPPED UP?

Balance, joint stability, and core training work are all interconnected. When you practice balance and joint stability exercises, you train your brain to quickly fire up and connect to all your peripheral muscles and nerves so that, if your balance is challenged, you are instinctively able to poise yourself.

To illustrate, let's use a real-life example. Suppose you are on an old, historic yet forgotten street in downtown Manhattan. Potholes are randomly scattered across the terrain. You are running late for work, as usual. Your cell phone is in one hand, and you're calling the office. Your mind is racing through a list of clever excuses to explain the delay, searching for an unused one. Your extra-hot morning coffee is in the other hand as you make an attempt to dash in front of the speedy bicycle messenger headed in your direction. You haphazardly take a step into a pothole.

Freeze right there. The good news is, if you've been working on core strength, balance, and joint stability training, the muscles that support your hips, ankles, and knees are strong and skilled, as are your core muscles. You'll likely able to avoid a nasty fall, a twisted ankle, a skin-blistering scald, or an unsightly stain on your freshly pressed white shirt. If you've not been working on anything but clicking the buttons on your remote control, or if you've been exercising but have not expanded your repertoire to include core, balance, and joint stability training, you and your shirt may be sharing that hot coffee.

Fine, so you don't live in a big city and you hate coffee. Well, do you ever ride the bus? Do you ever climb a ladder? Have you ever seen a banana peel on the floor? Do your kids leave their toys scattered all over the floor? There are endless opportunities for balance-challenging disasters, where your body would need to quickly adapt to a new environment in order to keep you standing. Core, balance, and joint stability training will help you to do so.

FLEXIBILITY

Consider this: Who will tie your shoes if you are not flexible enough to bend down and do it yourself? Will loafers one day be the only shoes inhabiting your California closet?

Independence is something to be carefully preserved. Being flexible will help you to maintain yours throughout your life. Flexibility is often defined as the range of motion around a joint or series of joints. In order to develop and maintain your flexibility, you must practice it, as any you do any other part of your fitness curriculum (for example, cardio and resistance). It is just as important.

If stretching is done correctly, it can help you avoid back pain while improving your posture, enable you to play sports better, and, overall, make you feel more like a teenager again. Your body will feel more free, flexible, and balanced. A little bit of Heaven on Earth!

> **THE LOWDOWN**
>
> **DAISY DUKES**
>
> Ladies: Don't plan a stretch session if you're wearing skimpy shorts or a mini-skirt. This could be embarrassing for everyone!

THE KICKBACKS

- Improves the quality of movement
- Increased range of motion
- Physical and mental stress buster
- Potential decrease of muscle aches, stiffness, and discomfort
- Helps support good posture
- Improves circulation

TRUTH BE TOLD

So, what are the common misconceptions about stretching? Check these out—as well as the more accurate information that follows.

MYTH: *I need to stretch before my workout.*

TRUTH Static, preworkout stretching is *not* a great idea. We generally recommend stretching *after* a workout, when increased blood flow through the muscles makes them warm and supple.

MYTH: *Stretching the muscle groups you are training in between sets is beneficial.*

TRUTH Actually, it is detrimental. The effectiveness of your next set may be decreased. Simply put, your first set primes your muscle so that it is more prepared to fire for the next. By stretching, you negate that effect to a certain degree.

MYTH: *I don't need to be flexible. My focus is on strength training.*

TRUTH Strength training and flexibility training should go hand in hand. A common misconception is that there must always be a trade-off between flexibility and strength. Don't focus on one to the detriment of the other. As a matter of fact, flexibility training and strength training can actually enhance each other.

MYTH: *Stretching will help create long, lean muscles.*

Good flexibility—and improved posture as a result—gives the appearance of looking longer and leaner, but muscles can't grow longer. Muscle tissue is lean tissue. To be "lean," you need to increase the ratio of muscle mass to body fat.

TRUTH

MYTH: *The more flexible I am, the better.*

For most, there is no reason to have the flexibility to put your feet behind your head. The point is to be flexible within a functional range of motion.

TRUTH

THE INSIDE SCOOP

- Don't leave it to instinct to tell you how to stretch properly. If stretching is done incorrectly, you could really hurt yourself. A great way to learn stretches and develop and practice your flexibility program is by taking Yoga or Stretch classes or by hiring a personal trainer.

- Before each stretch, take a deep breath. Imagine your breath going directly into the area you are about to stretch. Exhale and stretch to the point of noticeable but tolerable discomfort. (If you feel joint pain or as though you're about to tear something inside, ease up, and if the pain doesn't subside, *stop*.) Imagine the tension in your muscle being released with your breath and allow the muscle to adjust to this newly stretched position. Hold that stretch for about two seconds. Inhale as you release the stretch for another two seconds. Go back into the stretch, this time a bit deeper, and repeat. See Chapter 6 for a few examples of excellent stretches.

- If you are completely new to stretching, hire a professional certified trainer for a one-on-one stretch session. Don't let the look of it deceive you. Your trainer will have you in compromising positions. Not to worry; it is his or her job to do that, and you'll feel like a new person afterward.

TERMS OF "STRETCHOLOGY"

You'll come across a whole new vocabulary as you delve deeper into the practice of stretching. Some terms are safe and recommended, and others are dangerous and to be officially blacklisted from your stretch diaries. We'll describe a few of our favorite safe moves and also go over some potentially dangerous stretches. For a wonderfully user-friendly stretch resource, check out *Full Body Flexibility*, a book written by Jay Blahnik, a close friend and mentor.

Never bounce or make jerky movements during a stretch. This is called **ballistic stretching**, and should always be identified with the skull-and-crossbones symbol. It is using momentum of a moving part of the body in an attempt to force it to stretch beyond its normal range of motion. In this type of stretching, your muscles are jerked or bounced repeatedly into a position in an attempt to elongate them. Ballistic stretching is frowned upon as it can lead to injury. Because the muscles aren't given an opportunity to adjust and relax into the stretched position, they react in the opposite manner and tighten up. An example of ballistic stretching is bending at the waist and bouncing up and down in an attempt to touch your toes.

Dynamic stretching is not to be confused with ballistic stretching, although the two types of movement share a kindred connection. A dynamic stretch involves making controlled movements in an effort to increase mobility gradually. It requires extending the range of motion of those parts of the body being stretched to its limits, and never forcing it beyond. An example of dynamic stretching is a gentle and deliberate torso twist from one side to the other.

A **static stretch,** also sometimes referred to as a **passive stretch,** is one where a position is held using a part of the body, a stretching partner, or a piece of equipment. An example of this type of stretching is lying on the ground with one leg raised and using your hands to maintain that position in order to stretch the hamstring muscles. As your muscles acclimate to the stretching sensations, the notion is to ease yourself further into the stretch. If you are too aggressive with this type of stretching, it can also be dangerous. It is important not to push your stretch too far. Abusive static stretching joins ballistic stretching on the blacklist.

An **active stretch** differs from a static or passive stretch in that the position you assume is held in place using the strength of the opposing muscle group alone. For example, if you are trying to stretch the muscles of your chest, you would reach your arms back by engaging the muscles of the upper back.

Active-isolated stretching, commonly referred to as **AI stretching,** is highly regarded for its effectiveness and safety, and is a method often used by athletes, trainers, and massage therapists. It involves contracting the opposing muscle group, using your hands or a rope to assist the stretch, and holding the position for two-second intervals. These stretch intervals are bookended with equal periods of release. Stretches are meant to be gentle and unforced, and utilize the breath for best results. Breathe out during the stretch intervals and breathe in during the release periods.

Proprioceptive neuromuscular facilitation (PNF) is a partner-assisted flexibility technique combining muscle contraction and relaxation with passive and assisted stretching. It is known for its help in increasing range of motion. The idea is to push into the resistance provided by your partner in the opposite direction of the stretch, and then releasing. Upon releasing the contraction, the depth of the stretch is thought to be improved.

GROUP FITNESS CLASSES

4

Not less than two hours a day should be devoted to exercise, and the weather shall be little regarded. If the body is feeble, the mind will not be strong.

THOMAS JEFFERSON

THE VIRTUES OF GROUP FITNESS CLASSES

If you are just starting out, a group fitness class is a simple and effective way "in." This type of class functions like a personal training session but in a group setting. You don't need to do any preliminary preparation; the instructor does it all. He or she choreographs a balanced workout that is set to music; when the class is under way, the instructor is available to direct you and to give you tips and corrections on technique.

Are you familiar with the saying "there's power in numbers"? That certainly applies to group fitness classes. The energy flow created by the group dynamic acts as a source of motivation for you and makes the workout more fun for everybody. Within the group, you will also have an abundance of good examples from which to draw and learn. (Just be sure the instructor is doing his or her job and continually spot-checking the attendees to be sure they are doing the exercises correctly; follow the ones that seem to have the best form.) At the same time, with a group class, you blend in with the others so that you are not alone in the spotlight.

Because group fitness classes are scheduled for specific times, you need to mark down the schedules in your appointment book or whatever it is you use to keep track of your time. If you do so, you are much less likely to forget to go or want to skip the class. Having a set schedule eases the process of working out; you can simply fit the class into your natural routine and create a habit out of attending. When you are ready, the exercise routines you learn in class can be a great springboard for formulating your own private training sessions tailored to your personal needs.

THE LOWDOWN

ENERGY IS INFECTIOUS

A rigorous physical workout with a group of energetic people, along with the enthusiasm and motivation of an inspiring instructor, has been known to change people's lives. It can unearth a new and improved you from a body-mind-soul perspective, and give you a glimpse of the magnitude of your true potential.

PREEMPTIVE PECULIARITIES

Group fitness classes generally last from 30 minutes to one hour. They are normally broken down into three segments: the warm-up, the heart of the class, and the cool-down. The number of people in a group can vary greatly, but it usually tops off at approximately 40 people. We know, this sounds like a bit of a crowd, but larger exercise studios should be able to comfortably accommodate everyone. A trained instructor will guide and motivate the group through the class, usually with the help of carefully chosen tunes. Most of the time, the gym will provide any equipment required. The only things you will need to bring to every class are water and a towel.

If loud music irritates you, bring earplugs with you. A bit of toilet paper in each ear works quite effectively as well, although it will not score you any points on stylishness. Also look to position yourself away from the speakers.

If you are hypersensitive to temperature, dress in layers. As you warm up, peel off the outer clothes. (Please stop at the bottom layer!) If you have an aversion to breezes, do not pick a spot directly under a fan or in front of a vent. In most cases, the climate in a room will be appropriate for the type of workout you are doing.

Arrive early. Let the instructor know you are new to the class. Ask him or her if there is anything special you need to know about the class. Don't be shy. All questions are good ones. Asking them up-front will make you seem intelligent and could be a good way to get extra special attention during the class. Hey, you never know what can happen—the authors of this book met in class and ended up getting married!

THE LOWDOWN
SWEAT FACTOR

There are some who believe that the hotter the workout room, the more calories burned and the better the workout. Try not to fall into this erroneous mind-set. The heat generated during a workout and the resulting perspiration should come from your body engaging in the activity, not from the temperature of the room.

If you have any conditions you know may limit your ability to participate fully in any class (for example, pregnancy or an injury), let the instructor know before the start of class. Ask for suggested modifications.

Let the instructor know that you welcome feedback throughout the class. Getting some will speed up your learning curve and help you reach your goals more quickly.

WATER WORKS

Approximately 65 percent of an adult male's weight is made up of water. So, drink water not only before, during, and after a workout but all day long. It will prevent you from puffing up like a blowfish after a sodium-intense meal and keep you feeling fuller throughout the day. According to current German research, drinking cold water can help you burn extra calories. When you drink cold water, your body is prompted to generate more heat to maintain your normal body temperature. In doing so, it uses up more energy—that is, it burns calories. But drinking too much water in too short a period of time can be harmful as well. It may result in something called water intoxication, or *hyponatremia*. This condition is not something you should worry about, as it is a condition generally experienced by individuals who are doing some sort of long-distance endurance event like running a marathon.

Keep in mind: When first taking a class, it is perfectly fine to start slowly. Being overzealous and attempting the most advanced version of each exercise in the class could prove to be disastrous in many ways. You may disenchant yourself by not being able to keep up—and you could really hurt yourself. Progress only with the onset of confidence and comfort with the movements, and move on only as you build up your strength and endurance. Be diligent and patient with yourself.

Don't give up after one class. Don't be discouraged if it seems like you are the only one who does not know what you are doing. Everyone experiences his or her "first time" (in more ways than one). It's okay to not know exactly what you're doing the first few times. Give yourself at least three to four sessions in a class to begin to get a feel for it.

GIVE IT A CHANCE

Don't try a particular class four times in four years. To get a true feeling of what a class is all about, try to space the three-to-four-time tryout classes within a month or so.

You may find that you're particularly drawn to the basic concept of a class but aren't vibing with the instructor's style of teaching. If this is the case, don't immediately give that class the kiss of death and swear it off entirely. If you're fortunate enough to have the option of trying the same class with other instructors, you'll find that every instructor will infuse his or her own flavor to the class. Group fitness classes can be similar to shopping for sunglasses. Not every pair of shades will be right for every type of face. Some instructors' styles may work for your best friend but not for you. A large part of enjoying a class has to do with the instructor's personality and approach to fitness. It's important to try to find one that suits you and challenges you in just the right way.

If you have tried a class a number of times with several different instructors and still find that it just isn't your cup of tea, that's fine, too. There is no rule that says you must enjoy a seemingly popular class. As they say, different strokes for different folks.

Be an activist. Your comments are valuable to the managers of your gym. Once you get a feel for the class, share the good, the bad, and the ugly—and be specific. Your comments are the only way management can learn the ad hoc details of a class and are a great way to let management know that you would like to see more (or less) of those classes on the schedule. Your comments are also helpful to the individual instructors. Their periodic evaluations are mostly based on the consistent number of members they have in their classes and the comments that appear on the cards that members fill out.

THE "FAT-BURNING ZONE" IS NOT WHAT YOU PROBABLY THINK IT IS

The truth is, the higher the intensity of your workout, the more calories you burn and the more fat you burn. So, on the days you could be working hard, give it your all.

Here are some tips for getting the most out of your workout in class:

- In lieu of maneuvering yourself through a crowd of focused exercisers to get to the water fountain for a sip every 10 to 20 minutes, bring a water bottle with you to class.

- Avoid tripping accidents and keep the space around you free of clutter. Keep your hand weights, Body Bars, medicine balls, and the like, far from your stepping vicinity.

- Stand where you can clearly see your instructor, as well as other more experienced class takers, until you are comfortable with the class. Use others as role models.

- Being able to see yourself in the mirror is helpful as well. You will be able to visually check that you are doing the moves correctly.

The most popular classes tend to fill up long before the scheduled start of the class. Many gyms have found that the fairest solution to this problem is to have members sign up for those classes in advance. This is especially true of equipment-based classes such as Indoor Cycling, Urban Rebounding, BOSU, and Step. If you are planning on taking a class, be sure to ask someone at the front desk if you need to sign up and how long in advance you should arrive in order to guarantee getting a spot.

Do not walk into a class that is already in progress, especially if you have no previous experience with that class. In any case, if you are walking in late, be as inconspicuous as possible in setting up and joining in. The rule of thumb is that if the class has been going on for 10 minutes or longer, you're out of luck. You can choose to quietly sulk in the locker room, go home and eat bon-bons, or be a sport and try a different activity and plan to make it to another class—on time. Many gyms have strict rules about tardiness. With Cycling classes, some clubs may even stipulate that if you are not on your bike five minutes before the start of class, your bike will be up for grabs. Look for signs on the door or class schedule for information on the window of opportunity.

Explore the full gamut of classes available to you. Surely you will find a class or a few classes you particularly love. While this enthusiasm is a magnificent thing, we counsel you to take heed of falling into the pothole of doing only those classes. It is indispensable to keep your training diversified and to take a mélange of different types of classes. If you move your body in the same way, doing the same activity day in and day out, your body will eventually reach a plateau. Using the same muscles in the same ways over and over again without rest or variety will also prompt overuse injuries.

THE LOWDOWN

THE BROKEN RECORD

Think of a new compact disc you really enjoy listening to. At first, you anticipate listening to it over and over again, appreciating every note with emotional fulfillment. Even your neighbors, willingly or not, subconsciously memorize the lyrics to all your tunes. Let's call this the infatuation phase. After some time, the routine begins to get a bit tired and the thrill of it all is no longer as satisfying as it once was. Let's call this the real-life phase. You can no longer hear all of the intricacies you once appreciated and enjoyed so much. The CD may recognize your diminished esteem for it and begin to protest by skipping.

Your body will respond the same way as that once-beloved CD. The thing you once loved to do will become an agonizing routine and less interesting. Your muscles and joints, like the overused CD, may begin to protest and cease to cooperate. Their lack of cooperation, of course, will be interpreted in the form of injury and pain. Variety will keep you healthier and happier.

THE CLASS MENU

"Wow, that class looks like so much fun, but I could never do it." These are words we have heard a million times—and they are so often completely unwarranted. Looks can be deceiving. Through steam-covered windows and highly charged music, equally charged participants engaging in seemingly death-defying acts can make any class appear intimidating, almost frightening at first. The classes described in the paragraphs that follow are many of the most popular classes and some of the more cutting-edge ones being taught in gyms at present. We hope to dispel any fears or misconceptions you may have about these classes. We'll also share a little bit of history and cast light on what you can expect from a class, the fitness benefits associated with the activity, what to ask the instructor, and what to wear or bring to the session. Read on and you'll be prepared and brimming with confidence before you set foot in a new class.

Most group fitness classes will fit into one or more of the following categories:

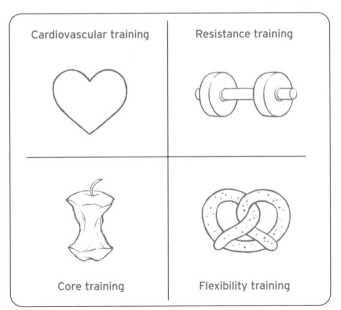

| Cardiovascular training | Resistance training |
| Core training | Flexibility training |

We've broken down the classes into these four categories using the symbols above. We highly recommend balancing your training by choosing classes that will allow you to benefit from all four categories.

ABS/CORE TRAINING CLASS

The main focus is on training the muscles of the core.

WHY CORE TRAIN?

The most obvious reason for taking this class is to develop increased core strength—the pillar supporting all other areas of strength. You will learn different ways to challenge your abs and lower back muscles. This is a great class for anyone.

THE INSIGHT

The importance of developing a strong core has given rise to a whole genre of classes. These classes focus strictly on strengthening the abdominal and lower back muscles, and usually last between 15 and 30 minutes. They are noteworthy for a couple of reasons.

Participating in such classes will ensure that you actually bestow upon your oft forgotten core muscles a spell of focused attention. Other classes may include a brief (usually 5- to 10-minute) period of core work at the beginning or end of the sessions, but because their main interests lie elsewhere, rarely do they dedicate enough time to provide you with a complete core workout. Just as with the training of all the other muscles in the body, training of the core muscles ought to be all-encompassing and varied in order to reap the best benefits. Taking classes will equip you with new techniques to keep your core training fresh and effective.

These classes are designed in many different ways, depending on the instructor. The most basic classes (note: *basic* does not mean *ineffective*) will be done standing or lying on an exercise mat for the duration of the class. Others will make use of a variety of supplementary equipment such as a Body Bar, a wedge, a BOSU, a medicine ball, or a Physio Ball. The options are limitless.

AEROBICS, HI-LO

Hi-Lo Aerobics are a combination of high-impact and low-impact moves in a choreographed, highly charged class format.

WHY HI-LO?

Hi-Lo Aerobics will strengthen your heart. These moves will increase coordination and mobility and invoke feelings similar to those associated with dancing. A Hi-Lo Aerobics class is fast-paced and lively.

While the high-impact moves may not be well suited for those suffering from joint ailments, they can be done with low-impact modifications, making this class appropriate for anyone.

THE CHRONICLES

Hi-Lo Aerobics class is a descendant of aerobic dance classes of the late 1960s. It became immensely popular in the early 1980s with the release of Jane Fonda's

workout video and book. Hi-Lo Aerobics still lives vigorously and in a variety of different versions today.

THE INSIGHT

Hi-ho, hel-lo. What are we talking here? As a group fitness neophyte, the title of the class is not very telling about what the class is going to be about. The "Hi" stands for high-impact, meaning that both feet will be required to lose contact with the floor at the same time. An example of a high-impact exercise is the well-known jumping jack. Conversely, the "Lo" stands for low-impact, meaning that at least one foot will maintain contact with the floor throughout the exer-

cise. An example of a low-impact move is a knee lift. In a nutshell, Hi-Lo Aerobics classes are a combination of choreographed high-impact and low-impact moves set to lively and energetic music.

There are many moves in a Hi-Lo Aerobics class that have rather strange names. You'll hear the instructor cuing moves like the grapevine, V-step, or box step. You'll be required to learn these steps, and it will take experiencing at least a couple of classes before you get used to them and the pace of the class. But be aware that there are only a handful of moves you'll need to learn, and once you get them down, you'll see that they're really not so complicated. Don't let the bouncy steps and fast pace put you off. Any of the moves of a Hi-Lo Aerobics class can be modified to be high-impact or low-impact. The choice is yours. Talk to the instructor before class. If you feel your joints are too delicate for all the leaping and bouncing high-impact moves, ask them to show you how to do the low-impact variations.

It is important to consider the level of intensity of a particular class before taking it. Ask the instructor about this as well. A beginner's class will teach you all the moves at a slower pace and emphasize repetition to allow you to get used to them. You'll find that struggling to keep up with your classmates is not very amusing, so avoid losing heart as a beginner and start learning with the beginners. Intermediate and advanced classes move much more quickly, and instructors often lead them with the assumption that the participants already know the basic moves and language, and will "jazz" them up with their own modifications and sequencing. The transitions from one move to the next will be speedy as well.

THE LOWDOWN

AEROBICS 101

- **Year 1968**—The word *aerobics* made its maiden voyage into the world of fitness. It was the title of a book written for the U.S. Air Force by a medical doctor named Kenneth Cooper. In this book, Cooper expressed his distress over the lack of physical activity and corresponding increased rates of heart disease in Americans. Aerobics was the term he used to denote the training system he prescribed to help remedy the situation. It was based on the idea that activities inducing prolonged stimulation of the heart and lungs would generate positive training effects in the body. "Aerobic" training, at the time, became a term mostly associated with running.

- **Year 1969**—Jacki Sorensen took Cooper's training to the next level by combining his training principles with ballroom and folk dancing moves and music. This marked the birth of "Aerobic Dancing." At the same time, Judy Sheppard Misset combined simple jazz dance moves with the aerobic concept and came up with "Jazzercise."

- **Year 1981**—This is the true beginning of it all. Jane Fonda published her first exercise video and book in 1981. The full-thigh-baring leotard, energetic music, and combination of high- and low-impact choreographed moves associated with her images propelled the "Aerobics" mass movement of the decade. Aerobics became known as the way to the "perfect body." Jane Fonda's videos and books were the first of the still extremely popular craze of celebrity exercise paraphernalia.

GROUP FITNESS CLASSES

To familiarize you with some of the universal Hi-Lo Aerobic terms you will encounter, we have listed and described a few of them below. Once again, don't let them scare you away. Once you get used to them, they will be a cinch to do.

The mother of almost all aerobics class moves is the grapevine. It is a lateral move that is so commonly used, it warrants a bit of further instruction. The sequence is as follows:

The Geapevine

1. Begin facing forward. Step to the side with your left foot.

2. Bring the right foot behind the left.

3. Step to the side with your left foot again.

4. Bring the right foot next to the left.

> From there the instructor will lead you into another move or repeat the grapevine in the opposite direction. Sometimes the sequence will end with a hamstring curl or a knee lift.

The March—Bring your knees toward your chest as you walk in place.

The V-Step—Step each foot wide out in front of you then bring them back together, tracing a "V" shape on the floor.

The Hamstring Curl—Lift your heel toward your butt.

The Knee Lift—Lift your knee up toward your chest.

The Repeater Curl—Several repetitions of kicking the same heel toward your butt.

The Repeater Knee—Several repetitions of lifting the same knee toward your chest.

The Jumping Jack—Stand with feet close together and arms down at your sides. Jump both feet out to the sides and raise both hands in an arc over your head. Jump again, and bring your feet and arms back to starting position. End softly by bending your knees a little as you land.

Hi-Lo Aerobics classes are traditionally floor-based and equipment-free. But in this day and age, there are many different takes on this class. For this reason, confirm with your instructor or a fellow class-taker whether any specific equipment will be needed for that particular class.

Much time has come to pass since the Jane Fonda days of high-cut leotards and leg warmers. Although this type of clothing is still functionally appropriate for Hi-Lo Aerobics class, better fashion judgment would suggest that you dress otherwise. Breathable, flexible, snug-fitting, and comfortable clothing coupled with a cross-training shoe is your best bet.

AEROBICS, STEP

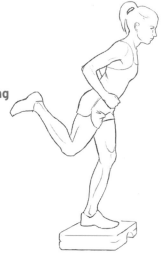

Step is a form of choreographed aerobic activity on an adjustable platform ranging from 4 inches to 10 inches in height.

WHY STEP?

Stepping will strengthen your heart and increase coordination and mobility. Similar to Hi-Lo Aerobics, stepping is fast-paced and lively, and will invoke feelings similar to those associated with dancing. All step moves can be modified to be low-impact and kind to the joints.

WOMAN DOING HAMSTRING CURL OFF A STEP.

THE CHRONICLES

Step classes took the nation by storm over a decade ago and have proven not to be a passing fad. They are still one of the most popular classes in the world, available in almost every gym known. The step moves are fascinating to watch, somewhat of a cross between a country line dance and a house party. The concept of Step

Aerobics was conceived by Gin Miller as a method of rehabilitation for her own personal knee injury. It was devised to be a new and improved form of aerobic exercise, minimizing the impact of the more traditional mixed high- and low-impact class.

THE INSIGHT

To the inexperienced, taking a Step class for the first time will feel somewhat like trying to get directions in Times Square in New York City when you're a visitor (yes, it's rough). The class has a language of its own. The names of the steps are completely unfamiliar to the nonstepper, and

your fellow stepping colleagues will be too busy trying to keep up with the choreography themselves to be able to translate. Basic Step, Over-the-Top, the Charleston Kick, and Around-the-World are just a few types of steps, and from them there are innumerable variations.

A Step class is different from the traditional Hi-Lo class in that each person works within his or her own space surrounding the platform. If you are new to stepping, find out if your gym offers a beginners class that will introduce you to the very basic steps with easier-to-follow combinations. Start with that. As a beginner, also start with a low platform. As you get better at the steps and get used to them, move up in the world and take it up another riser. When you get really good and are looking for a bigger challenge, add "power" to your moves. You do that by getting some air on the way up. The moves then become high-impact, where both feet are off the Step at the same time.

THE LOWDOWN

STELLAR STEPPING STRATEGY

Pay attention to your alignment. Look proud. Keep your head up and chest lifted. Push your shoulders down and back, and brace your core (abdominal muscles).

Make sure your foot is in the center of the platform and your heel is down. If you do so, you will avoid injury to the Achilles tendon (the tendon that attaches the base of your heel to your calf).

Each time you step down, do so fully and close to the platform. Come down toe-ball-heel, allowing your heels to touch the floor. Doing so will help absorb shock.

The only time you will be on the balls of your feet is when you are doing lunges or repeater steps. In these cases, your weight should be on the working leg and your heel of the nonworking leg off the floor.

Don't use hand or leg weights when stepping. The possibility of injury outweighs the benefits of adding weight.

For the conventional Step class, you will only need your Step and your own personal pool of energy to draw from in order to participate in class. To step out in style, consider outfitting yourself as you would for a Hi-Lo class. Since you will be repeatedly stepping on and off the platform, wearing extra long and wide bottomed pants may prove to be awkward and accident-inducing. Consider the old Bon Jovi album *Slippery When Wet* as cautionary counsel and bring a towel to wipe the sweat off yourself and your Step.

THE LOWDOWN

THE SUPER STEP

The Step, as a piece of equipment, is quite versatile, and is sometimes used in Body Conditioning or Sculpt classes as a bench or platform on which to do resistance training and abdominal work. For those classes, the Step is the auxiliary equipment and you will need to ask your instructor for more information on what else may be needed.

AQUA AEROBICS CLASSES

These classes take place within a pool. Unless the class is described as a straightforward swim class on your schedule, it will most likely have nothing to do with actual swimming. It will be geared toward providing in-water, minimal-impact cardiovascular training, with perhaps an element of resistance training.

WHY AQUA AEROBICS?

Aqua Aerobics classes will strengthen your heart (class with a cardio focus), increase strength and flexibility, and help tone your muscles. Water supports your body and makes exercise feel easier. It also provides buoyancy, which helps to protect the joints and makes aqua workouts low-impact. Plus, playing in the water is fun and safe for all.

THE CHRONICLES

In the interest of finding ways to soften the impact of the more traditional high-impact aerobic exercise in the 1990s, aqua aerobics was born.

THE INSIGHT

The primary mission of an aqua aerobics workout is to improve cardiovascular conditioning in a way that is not overly demanding on the joints, bones, and muscles. While submerged in water your body is only responsible for supporting 10 to 15 percent of its body weight while the rest of your weight is protected by the buoyancy and support of water. As a result, during your water workout you'll gain all the cardiovascular benefits associated with aerobic exercise on dry land, but with only a fraction of the amount of stress to your joints, bones, and muscles. This feature makes aqua aerobics an awesome alternative for anyone who is joint sensitive or arthritic, overweight, pregnant, recovering from surgery or injury, or sedentary and looking to begin an aerobic conditioning program. Please make sure to seek approval from your physician before beginning any type of workout program.

In addition to healthy joints, bones, and muscles, developing a semi-aquatic workout lifestyle will provide many additional health benefits for you. One such benefit is muscle strength. Have you ever tried to run underwater? If you have, you know that it's nearly impossible to move your legs with any speed. Water offers resistance that will help strengthen your muscles as you move in opposition to it. Another benefit involves flexibility. You'll be amazed by your ability to stretch underwater. Water has the effect of nullifying the impact of gravity. This effect will also allow you to engage in stretches you may have otherwise considered impossible on land.

And now the questions: What exactly will you be doing while immersed in a pool of water in aqua aerobics? Is having the ability to swim a prerequisite? What are the odds of drowning during vigorous activity? Should you wear a life jacket? If you've been led to believe that aqua aerobics is in any way related to the inverted water dance loved by Esther Williams' fans, synchronized swimming, or water ballet, you have been wickedly misguided. Aqua Aerobics classes, as all other aerobics-based classes, are generally 45 to 60 minutes long, are set to music, and incorporate a variety of dance like steps or calisthenics-type moves. The distinguishing factor is that these moves are all performed while your body is underwater. Fear not, you won't need an aqualung to benefit from this class. You'll usually work out in shallow water that reaches to your waist or to your chest. With any deeper-

delving exception, you'll be equipped with a flotation device. Some classes may require the use of water-appropriate hand weights and kickboards and will incorporate a resistance training component into the program.

Swimming may or may not be a part of the class agenda. Be candid with your instructor about your swimming abilities and feelings about working out in water. The class may be structured to be a salutary influence on you regardless of your involvement in the swimming aspect of the class.

THE LOWDOWN

AQUATIC CALORIE KINDLING

Are the calorie-blasting benefits of an Aqua Aerobics class comparable to those of a dry class? Generally, because of the diminished effects of gravity underwater, and its ability to support such a large percentage of your weight, you won't burn as many calories pool-entrenched as if you did the same workout poolside, in the same amount of time.

Not surprisingly, acceptable aqua-tire differs from other gym garb. Most gyms will not allow anything but the full swimsuit–swim cap combination in the pool. Water shoes are often not required, but also a good idea. They'll protect your tootsies from cuts and scrapes from gravelly pool floors. If the class composition entails swimming, you may also want to adorn your eyes with the proper protection and invest in a pair of goggles. Any other necessary equipment will be provided by the gym.

BODY CONDITIONING OR BODY SCULPT

A broad spectrum of classes with the common aim of shaping, toning, and defining the muscles.

WHY BODY SCULPT?

Body Sculpt is a great way to increase muscle strength and endurance. A Body Sculpt class is relatively slow paced and easy to follow, and is the closest thing to a free personal training session—and we all like "free," don't we?

THE CHRONICLES

In the 1980s Jane Fonda began a fitness movement through her aerobics-based group classes, book, and exercise video. With the growing recognition of the value of resistance training in a balanced fitness program, Body Sculpt classes were the natural progression. Today, Body Sculpt classes are all the rage and you'll find at least one version of this type of class at just about any fitness facility in the world.

THE INSIGHT

There is a vast array of creative class titles that all fall under the Body Conditioning or Body Sculpt umbrella. Don't be frightened by wild-sounding class names on your schedule. The main objective of these classes is to increase muscle endurance and strength. Increasing muscle strength will heighten the rate at which your body uses energy (burns calories) both while you are working out and while your body is at rest. Any type of weight training exercise will also help to maintain or increase bone density and ward off the prospect of osteoporosis in later years. These classes are a great way to learn basic resistance training exercises that can later be used on the training floor. Having a strong body will enable you to feel free and function comfortably throughout your life.

As many different names as there are for body conditioning classes, there may be an even greater number of tools or equipment used in these classes. For example, in any one class you may need a Body Bar, a medicine ball, BOSU, hand weights, and Dyna-Bands.

GROUP FITNESS CLASSES

CONDITIONING BY ANY OTHER NAME . . .

Some examples of "creative" sounding classes that are really forms of Body Sculpt classes are Recess, Ballistic Body, Diesel, Final Cut, Liquid Strength, Body Pump, Brazilian Butt Lift, Sweat, Band Camp, Jump and Pump.

Many Body Sculpt classes will incorporate several different pieces of equipment into the workout. Some will have you moving from station to station, each one focusing on a different piece of equipment and a different body part or body function. These types of classes often provide a great introduction to equipment that is new to you, perhaps one you grow to love and integrate into your own personal workouts as you get more comfortable. Call it an easy first date. There's no commitment, you need to dedicate only a short time span, and you can get to know each other through the guidance of a professional. Many Body Sculpt classes incorporate cardio intervals into the workout. For example, they may make use of the rebounder, BOSU, or jump rope, among other tools as stations in a circuit class. Keep in mind: If after reading our synopsis of the Urban Rebounding and BOSU classes, mentioned later, you're still unsure about your ability to master the equipment, a Sculpt class utilizing those pieces of equipment may be a good icebreaker.

One of the big misconceptions surrounding body sculpting is that if you "lift weights" you will end up looking like Arnold Schwarzenegger in his heyday. Be reassured that growing to a massive bodybuilder's size or anything close to it is almost a full-time job. It takes very heavy weight lifting, a huge amount of time, hard work, unyielding dedication, and a good dose of testosterone to add that type of mass to your frame. The 5- to 12-pound weights and the high number of repetitions usually required in a Sculpt class will do what they say they will— *sculpt* your muscles. If you're looking to gain muscle mass, don't look to a Sculpt class. Get out on the training floor and hire a trainer. In order to reap those benefits, be prepared to pay the price.

Before taking a Sculpt class for the first time, be sure to ask the instructor what the focus of the class will be. Sculpt classes could be focused on muscle endurance, muscle strength, or a combination of both. Some classes will target isolated muscle groups such as the lower body or upper body. Knowing what the focus of the class will be will help you determine whether you will need heavier weights, lighter weights, or a variety of different types of weights.

WEIGHTY DECISIONS

- Muscle endurance—Higher repetitions (12 to 20), lighter weight

- Muscle strength—Lower repetitions (8 to 12), heavier weight

How do you know if you have the right weight for a particular exercise?

After completing a full set, you should feel like you have noticeably and genuinely fatigued the muscle group you are working. You'll feel a moderate to high level of discomfort in the form of burning. If you finish the set and feel like you are able to squeeze out another 6 to 10 reps, and if you're interested in results, go with a heavier weight the next time.

If at any point during the set your form falters, consider switching to lighter weights. For example, if you have to shrug your shoulders up to your ears or use momentum in order to lift the weight, lighten your load.

Want a few pointers? The following will help you get started.

Your core should be braced during all exercises. Your core muscles will stabilize and support your lower back. How do you brace your core? Imagine the sides of your stomach are being vigorously tickled. Bracing would be your instinctive reaction. Perhaps you are not ticklish. In this case, imagine you are being punched in the stomach. In order to ward off the blow, you would naturally brace your core. While bracing, you should still be able to breathe comfortably.

Keep your shoulders down and locked into your back. How? Start by bringing your shoulders all the way up to your ears. Roll your shoulders, like a wave, down and back. Hold this position. Your neck should feel long and your chest open and proud.

Keep your neck aligned with your spine and never pushed forward (like a pecking chicken).

A few very important exercises that will most likely make their way into any Body Conditioning or Sculpt class are push-ups, squats, and lunges. They are basic and very functional exercises because they collectively target multiple muscle groups. They also require a little bit of guidance and practice to perfect.

PUSH-UP

The **push-up** will work your pectoral muscles (chest), anterior deltoids (front part of your shoulders), triceps (back of the upper arm), and quadriceps (front of your thighs), in addition to challenging your core stabilization. Here is how to do one correctly.

Kneel on the floor with your hands wider than shoulder width apart and your fingers angled in toward each other slightly. Brace your core muscles and straighten your legs so that you are in a straight line from the top of your head to your toes. Bend your elbows to about 90 degrees, lowering the middle of your chest toward the floor directly in between your hands. Imagine you are pushing the floor away from you to return to starting position. If a full push-up is too difficult, try doing one from your knees.

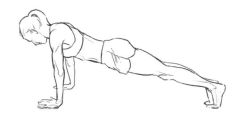
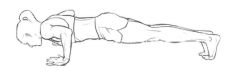

A PERFECT PUSH-UP SHOULD LOOK LIKE THIS. YOUR BODY SHOULD BE IN A STRAIGHT LINE FROM THE TOP OF YOUR HEAD TO YOUR TOES THROUGHOUT THIS EXERCISE.

THE LOWDOWN

POLITE PUSH-UP

Save the pelvic thrust for your Britney Spears impersonation. This is an ineffective way to do a push-up.

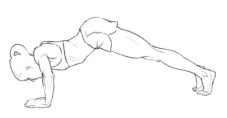
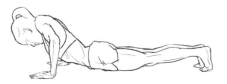

PROBLEM PUSH-UPS: IN THE TOP ILLUSTRATION, THE BUTTOCKS ARE TOO HIGH IN THE AIR AND THE BODY IS ARCHED; IN THE BOTTOM ILLUSTRATION, THE LOWER PART OF THE BODY IS TOO LOW TO THE GROUND.

SQUAT

The **squat** will work your quadriceps, hamstrings, and gluteals (thighs, hips, and butt), and will also fire up the core muscles as stabilizers. Here is how to do one correctly: Stand with your feet approximately hip to shoulder width apart. Bend your knees and push your hips back as you lower your body down as far as you can, up to a 90-degree angle. You should feel your weight directly over your ankles. Keep your chin lifted off your chest and your focus out in front of you. Imagine pushing the ground away from you with your feet as you stand up to starting position.

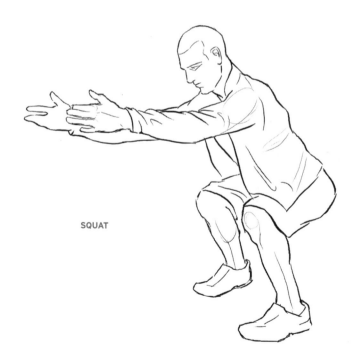

SQUAT

LUNGE

The **lunge** is essentially a split squat. It will work your quadriceps, hamstrings, and gluteals (thighs, hips, and butt) and will also fire up the core muscles as stabilizers. Here is how to do one correctly: Stand with your feet approximately shoulder width apart. Take a large step forward in a straight line. Your weight should be evenly distributed between both feet. This is your starting position. Keeping your torso upright, bend both knees and lower your hips straight down toward the floor.

Most of your weight should now be over the ankle of your front leg and your back heel will be off the floor. Your front knee should be bent up to 90 degrees. Imagine you are pushing the floor away with your feet to return to starting position.

Keep your body weight back. Your knees should never extend beyond your toes when doing a squat or lunge of any sort. This may eventually negatively affect your knees.

The proper attire for Body Conditioning classes is basically anything that feels comfortable to move around in. Any type of training shoe will work as well. As usual, it is wise to have a towel and water handy.

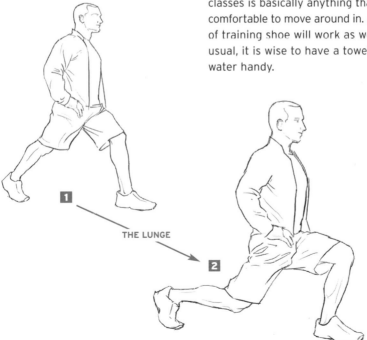

THE LUNGE

BOOT CAMP CLASS

An intense off shoot of a Body Conditioning class fusing military-based moves.

WHY BOOT CAMP?

Boot Camp is an advanced basic-training-inspired class that will strengthen your heart and is a great way to increase muscle strength and endurance.

THE CHRONICLES

Old-school boot camp, as a means to weed out true civilians from those destined to become mean, lean warriors, has been around for quite some time. As a recreational means of giving chase to a more fit body, however, it is a fairly new innovation, making its way into the limelight in the mid- to late 1990s. These classes first sprouted up as private 6- to 12-week courses, usually taking place outdoors, and run by true ex-military members. These days, various renditions of group fitness classes based on boot camp practices find their homes in gyms everywhere.

THE INSIGHT

As the name implies, Boot Camp is intended to emulate actual military basic training. This training is usually meant to be advanced. The military aspect of this class stems from the idea of going through a chain of exercises strung together with little to no rest in between, as well as the idea of working in a team and fostering the spirit of camaraderie. The basic training you will get in Boot Camp classes (no pun intended) will be a multifaceted series of plyometric, calisthenic, endurance, cardiovascular, and resistance training drills and more. You may be running, kickboxing, going through obstacle courses, and doing sit-ups and push-ups, among other things, either alone, with a single partner, or with a larger team. Essentially, anything goes in this type of class.

PLYO-PONDER

What is a plyometric exercise? Have you ever watched sprinters in action and wondered how they're able to run so fast? Their legs practically blur before your eyes. Plyometric training is what helps develop fast-twitch muscle fibers. What exactly is it? Think of stretching out a coiled spring as far as possible and then letting it go. In the fraction of a second it takes for the spring to recoil, explosive energy is released. In the same way, a muscle is able to contract with a greater amount of strength and speed if it is first quickly lengthened. Plyometric exercises are quick, explosive, jumping drills that work to help the muscles develop the ability to rapidly and vigorously lengthen and recoil.

The makeup of a Boot Camp class will really depend on the instructor. Check out how a few different instructors orchestrate their classes. Boot Camp classes are usually meant for the more conditioned individual. A great thing to ask the instructor before taking class is if the class accommodates participants at your level.

If camouflage is your thing, feel free to sport your military gear in Boot Camp class. The class dress code, however, is far less stringent than that of the military. Slip into something unrestricting and comfortable to move around in. Any type of training shoe will work, but a cross-training shoe is recommended. It will give you extra support, especially when doing lateral (side-to-side) movements. You'll definitely need to towel off and keep hydrated during class, so bring a towel and water.

BOSU

While the BOSU may appear to be an alien-like space pod, it is actually a handy apparatus with great versatility. A BOSU is a rubber, dome-shaped, air-filled pod used as a tool to add balance challenges to otherwise basic exercises. BOSU stands for "both sides up" because it can be used with the dome side up or the platform side up. A BOSU class will predominantly focus on training with the BOSU, and may or may not also use other equipment.

WHY BOSU?

Working on the unstable surface of the BOSU encourages increased joint stability and will increase your coordination and balance. It is a low-impact workout that is appropriate for all ages.

Because a BOSU enhances the efficiency of your neuromuscular connection, it is a "smart-body" workout.

THE CHRONICLES

The importance of balance in all facets of movement became clear to David Weck of San Diego, California, while he was working to overcome his own back problems. A vision of a device to improve balance resulted in the conception of the BOSU Balance Trainer. The first prototype was tested on a group of professional and Olympic teams in 1999 to a no-less-than-staggering reaction. Through the athletic grapevine, news of the BOSU spread, and Weck's first major sale of the BOSU went to the U.S. Ski Team. He continues to work with the team today.

THE LOWDOWN
CLOWNING AROUND

"I really love the Bozo class. It really challenges my core muscles in a different way." A friend of ours would say this to us after every BOSU class she took. No matter how many times we corrected her, we could not get her to say say "Bow-Sue" (as it is correctly pronounced). Maybe it is because she felt like a Bozo trying to balance on the BOSU during class. Whatever it was, she was a regular in class and we love her for her unique pronunciation.

GROUP FITNESS CLASSES

THE INSIGHT

The air-filled dome of the BOSU acts as an unstable surface, so any move performed on it (even simply standing up), becomes much trickier than it ordinarily would be. A BOSU class can be focused on anything from basic balance and stabilization to cardiovascular, resistance, and core training. The experience of working on the BOSU will be different from working on any other piece of equipment and you'll feel sensations in places you wouldn't expect. For example, you'll feel discomfort in the arches of your feet. They will feel as if they were trying to grab on to the BOSU. This sensation is absolutely normal. Your feet are working to adapt to the new unstable surface and are trying to help you maintain your balance. This sensation will dissipate and become more tolerable over time.

BOSU classes may make you feel a bit like a Bozo in the beginning because you are unfamiliar with the mechanics of keeping your balance on the unstable surface. But never fear, the BOSU class is one of the least intimidating you'll find at the gym.

Reservations about using the BOSU are commonly based on a fear of looking silly or goofy in front of strangers. In this case, the BOSU can double as your psychotherapist, helping you work through that source of anxiety. The objective of working on the BOSU is to increase your coordination, balance, and overall body awareness. In order to reach this objective, your sense of balance and stability is sometimes provoked to the point where it is virtually lost, requiring you to recenter yourself. This experience, in a BOSU class, is a good thing. It's a sign that you are challenging yourself at a level that will bring positive results.

Another common concern with the BOSU has to do with the fear of falling off. If you're uncomfortable with height, keep in mind: when standing on the BOSU, your feet will be less than a foot off the ground. If you lose your balance, all you have to do is step off.

THE LOWDOWN

SPATIAL SMARTS

If you're working with hand weights or any other equipment in a BOSU class, keep everything you're not using at that moment far enough away from the BOSU so that you have room to step off, if you need to. You don't want to trip on anything if you lose your balance.

Everyone's sense of balance is inconsistent. Some days we feel rooted and others we're off kilter. This variation is because your sense of balance is so closely related to so many things, for example, how tired you are, if you are feeling sick, and if you are in a bad mood. On those off-kilter days, when doing work on the BOSU is more distracting than beneficial, do the tricky moves on the floor. Sight plays a very important role in balance and stability: on a day you're feeling very balanced, try standing on the BOSU with your eyes closed.

When a newcomer is first taking a BOSU class, one of the biggest challenges is to find the right position. Be proactive in

resituating yourself until you find the most stable position. Most importantly, be patient; everything will come together and your body will develop new coordination strategies as it adjusts to the mechanics of the BOSU.

The best footwear for working on the BOSU is a cross-training shoe. The narrow base and elevated heel characteristic of running shoes will increase the challenge many-fold. To avoid slipping off the BOSU during seated or lying work, dress in snug-fitting clothing made of nonslippery fabric. You will need to have a towel with you for class. Sweat on the surface of the BOSU will sometimes make it slippery and difficult on which to work. Be sure to keep hydrated as well.

For all you women fashion divas, this is the secret weapon for walking gracefully and elegantly in your favorite four-inch heels. Working on the BOSU will strengthen all your joints, especially your ankles, knees, and hips. Your catwalk will look smooth, stylish, and easy. For sports enthusiasts and athletes not necessarily concerned about their abilities on stilettos, the BOSU is an indispensable tool for improving motor skills.

BOXING

Boxing classes, which are based on the principles of the sport, may or may not employ traditional boxing equipment such as a speed bag, heavy bag, jump rope, and boxing gloves.

WHY BOX?

Boxing is a fantastic full-body workout. It will challenge your heart while toning your muscles and improving your speed, agility, and coordination. It's also a fantastic way to release pent-up aggression.

THE CHRONICLES

Boxing, as a sport, has survived the test of time. It can be traced back as far as ancient Greece, where it made up part of the Olympic Games. In the eighteenth century, it became a popular sport in England, but really established itself as a working-class pastime and sport favorite during the Industrial Revolution. As a group fitness class, Boxing emerged in the 1990s.

THE INSIGHT

Engaging in any professional sport on an amateur, nonthreatening level is a wonderful experience. This can be said of Boxing classes as well. It's one of the most effective total-body workouts, combining cardiovascular, resistance, agility, and coordination training components. Some facilities will provide a full-on boxing experience. You'll wear those padded gloves sported by the pros, punch the same types of bags as boxers do during their training, and learn all of the fancy foot, punching, and dodging techniques. Some classes will even take place within a boxing ring. Other Boxing classes are more deeply committed to providing a boxing-esque experience, with a stronger focus on cardiovascular conditioning. You may or may not be gloved up, and may or may not be punching boxing bags. What you will be doing is learning boxing-like moves and training principles, and reaping the heart-felt and auxiliary muscle toning benefits.

The dress code for Boxing classes is like that of other group fitness classes, so show up wearing breathable, flexible, and comfortable clothing. Boxing demands a certain amount of footwork, often with

lateral movement. For this reason, that good, old wide-based cross-training shoe works very well for this class. If you're so inclined, you could also spring for a true boxing shoe, which generally has a flat sole, and a higher top that wraps around the ankle for additional support. If the class you're taking requires boxing gloves, your gym will most likely provide them. You'll also need wraps, which are worn under boxing gloves for extra support of the wrists and fists. These wraps, however, will not be furnished for you. For that, you should be grateful. Wraps tend to get sweaty, and sweaty palms are never pleasant. Just imagine having to box with your hands wrapped in someone else's sweaty palms.

GROUP FITNESS CLASSES

CAPOEIRA

Dance- and martial arts–infused class based on the art originating in Brazil.

WHY CAPOEIRA?

Capoeira will strengthen your heart by providing an intense aerobic workout. It will help increase flexibility, balance, coordination, and reflexes. Capoeira is a great way to reduce stress, boost your fitness level, and strengthen your mind-body connection while at the same time developing some impressive acrobatic skills.

> **THE LOWDOWN**
>
> ### SAY IT RIGHT
> The correct pronunciation of the word *Capoeira* is *Ka-pu-era*. Say it slowly and loudly to yourself in front of a mirror at home 10 times and you will be good to go.

THE CHRONICLES

You can usually hear the sounds of a berimbao (a long stick-like instrument specific to the art) and chanting long before you will be able to see a group of people practicing Capoeira. What exactly is it? It's a spirited, acrobatic, and powerful art form, and simultaneously a graceful and flowing dance. It is based on a self-defense technique developed by slaves brought to Brazil from Angola in the sixteenth century. The slaves masked their practice by making it look like harmless dance so that the slave masters would not know that they were, in fact, combat training. Capoeira was officially banned in Brazil even after slavery was abolished but continued to be secretly practiced by the poorer population. In the 1930s the cultural value of Capoeira was finally recognized and the ban was lifted. It is the second most popular sport in Brazil (second to fútbol, or soccer, of course) and is slowly gaining popularity all over the world.

THE INSIGHT

Capoeira, as a group fitness class, is adapted from the historic Brazilian art, and the moves you will be learning will combine martial arts and dance. You will be taught the rhythm and strategy of Capoeira and the various kicks, ducks, turns, and punches associated with it. It is a dynamic and challenging heart-throbbing workout, and it will undoubtedly help build strength and endurance.

We can see how there may be many qualms about trying this class. Even its name is rather unusual. Simply being able to pronounce the name correctly may dare your tongue to maneuver itself in new and exciting ways. What about the rest of the body? The idea of sparring is rarely one that paints an inviting picture. For the majority of the population, adding the element of dance to the mix may be enough for anyone to add Capoeira to their list of things to steer clear of.

Practicing Capoeira is called playing, because it is really not meant to be a violent activity. The participants may look like they are fighting, but never actually strike or touch each other. As you can imagine, this requires plenty of experience and control. Because of this, in a group fitness class at a gym, you will be learning the moves and practicing them to Afro-Brazilian beats, but will not actually be sparring. If you sign up for classes outside of a gym, this may not be true. Check with that specific facility.

This is an equipment-free class. Bring only yourself and your comfortable clothing with you in order to participate. You want to be able to move around comfortably without getting tangled up in excess fabric. Your particular gym may or may not require you to wear shoes, so peek into a class before trying it or ask the instructor whether shoes are necessary.

CARDIO KICKBOXING

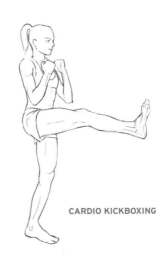

Cardiovascular training that combines boxing and martial arts techniques.

WHY CARDIO KICKBOX?

Cardio Kickboxing class will strengthen your heart and is a great way to increase muscle strength and endurance. At the same time, you'll learn a new skill and get a taste of self-defense training.

CARDIO KICKBOXING

THE CHRONICLES

Kickboxing finds its roots in martial arts, in the practices of ancient warriors of Asian countries such as Korea, Japan, China, and Thailand. Kickboxing, as a sport, is a concept that was developed in the United States in the 1970s.

It combines the kicking and punching techniques of eastern martial arts with that of western boxing. Cardio kickboxing incorporates kickboxing kicks, punches, and blocks into a workout.

THE INSIGHT

The benefits of this type of training are extensive. An hour-long class will give you a hearty cardiovascular workout, and in addition you'll be building endurance, strength, and flexibility, toning your muscles, improving balance and coordination, and sharpening your reflexes.

There is a certain sense of power that comes from kicking and punching. It's a great way to improve your self-defense skills and also an excellent way to liberate any pent-up anger you may have developed during the day.

Unless you're opposed to using keys and prefer to kick open doors, many of the moves in a Kickboxing class won't be familiar to you. They're also not the types of moves you would encounter in other group fitness classes. This can be scary and may cause you to shy away from taking this class. For this reason, we went ahead and put together a list of basic kickboxing moves, along with nifty pointers that were given to us by Violet Zaki, a kickboxing guru who happens to be a great friend of ours. Read our guidelines and trade in your fears for a fierce new self-defending body. (For more information on Violet, visit www.zakifitness.com.)

CARDIO KICKBOXING RULES OF THUMB

Pay attention to your body. Don't do anything that doesn't feel right to you, even if you're doing it correctly. What we mean by this is that you should not feel pressured to punch faster or kick higher than you are safely able to. Having arthritis, tight hamstrings, or an inflexible back may make cardio kickboxing a bit more challenging for you. Take it easy on yourself. Your speed, endurance, and flexibility will get better with practice.

Do not wear leg or arm weights or hold dumbbells when you're punching or kicking. The increased risk of joint injury far outweighs any added benefits.

Do not overextend your kicks. Kick only as high as you can raise your leg while maintaining proper body alignment.

Do not lock your joints when kicking and punching.

Always keep your eyes on your opponent and your chin up!

General punching tips:

- Keep your wrists straight and strong.

- Use the first two knuckles for striking.

- Always look at where your punches are going.

- Use your body weight to throw a power punch. Keep your shoulders lined up by pivoting your feet, rotating your hips, and using your thighs.

BASIC POSITIONS

GUARD POSITION Your fists are in line and slightly under your chin. Keep your elbows pointing down.

FIGHTING POSITION This is the starting position for all kickboxing moves. Stand with your feet on a diagonal approximately shoulder width apart. Your front foot should be flat with your toe pointing forward, while you will be on the ball of your back foot. Your weight should be evenly distributed. Keep your knees slightly bent and your hands in guard position. Engage your abs.

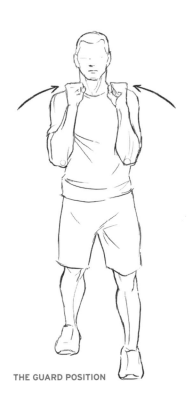

THE GUARD POSITION

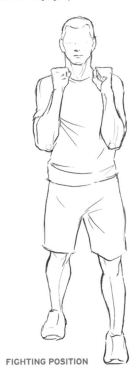

FIGHTING POSITION

! **WHEN YOU LOOK INTO A MIRROR, YOU SHOULD BE ABLE TO SEE BOTH FEET COMPLETELY**

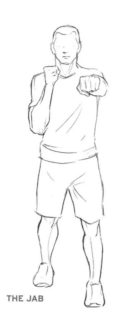

THE JAB

THE PUNCHES

THE JAB From fighting position, extend the same arm as your forward foot straight out in front of you while turning your fist so that your palm faces the ground at the point of contact. Once your arm is fully extended, tuck the elbow in to immediately bring it back to starting position. When you extend your arm, keep your shoulders and hips aligned and do not lock your elbow.

> **!** DO NOT LET YOUR ELBOW SWING OUT. KEEP YOUR BODY BALANCED THROUGHOUT THE JAB. IF YOU ARE LOOKING IN A MIRROR, YOU WILL BE AIMING TOWARD YOUR NOSE.

THE CROSS This punch comes from the rear arm from fighting position. Begin by rotating your back hip forward and pivoting your back foot. Your power will come from the pivot movement of the body. Line up your back shoulder with your target. Extend your arm and turn your fist so that your palm faces the ground at the point of contact. Once your arm is fully extended, bring it immediately back to starting position.

> **!** DO NOT MOVE YOUR ARMS FIRST. THE FIRST MOTION SHOULD BE THE TURNING OF YOUR BODY.

Do not bend from the hips.

Push off the ground with your back foot.

Keep your knee and toe lined up.

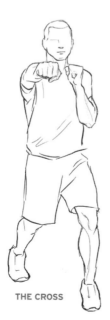

THE CROSS

THE HOOK From fighting position, lift the elbow and rotate your shoulder, hip, and back foot in the direction of your target. Your heel lifts slightly as you strike. Use the rotation of your body to add power and momentum to your blow.

THE UPPERCUT With arms in guard position, bring your fist back to your shoulder and down to your hip while turning your palm up. As you drop your hand, your torso will turn with the punch and your shoulders will drop. Keep your knees slightly bent. Move your arm upward, with your palm facing your chest, and stop at the chin. Pivot your foot and hip slightly as you do this. This will give power to your punch.

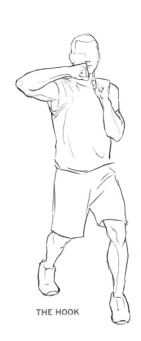

THE HOOK

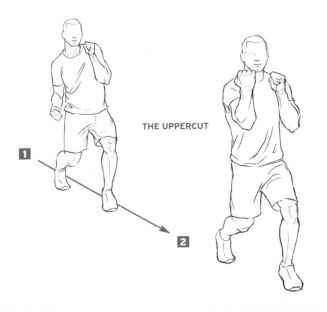

THE UPPERCUT

DEFENSIVE MOVES

THE DUCK The duck is a modified squat. All the rules for performing a squat correctly apply here as well, except that you should not go deeper than a quarter of the way down when using this in a combination.

THE SHIN BLOCK You are basically using your shin to protect your body from getting hit by doing a knee lift. Engage your abs tightly and squeeze the gluteal muscles of the rear leg. Keep your shoulders facing forward and your arms in guard position. Lift your knee to the center of the chest. Keep your toes pointed and your heel close to your hamstrings.

> **!** DO NOT BRING YOUR CHEST DOWN TO MEET YOUR KNEE; BRING YOUR KNEE TO YOUR CHEST.

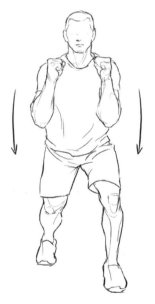

THE DUCK

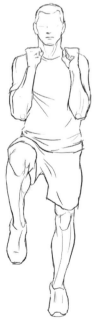

THE SHIN BLOCK

THE KICKS

THE FRONT SNAP KICK From fighting position, aim and raise your knee to your target and extend your leg. Keep your toes pointed. Keep your shoulders engaged and in front of your hips to help maintain balance. This can be done with the front or rear leg as the kicking leg.

THE FRONT THRUST KICK This is the same as the snap kick, except your foot is flexed so that you are using your heel to kick. Imagine you are trying to kick open a locked door.

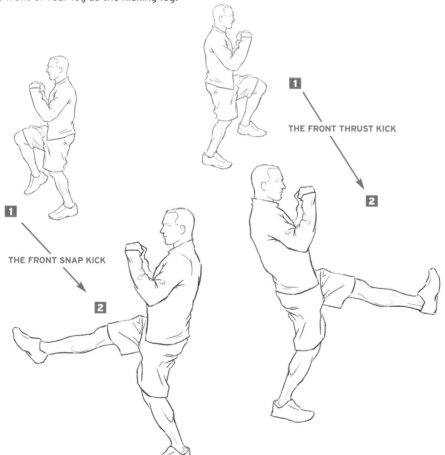

THE FRONT THRUST KICK

THE FRONT SNAP KICK

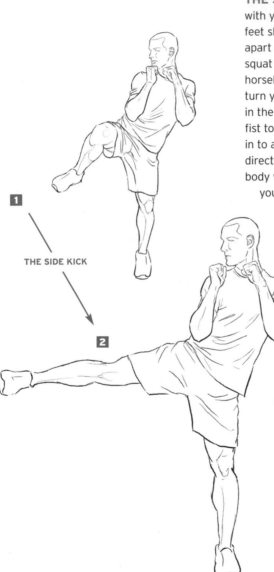

THE SIDE KICK

THE SIDE KICK Stand facing forward with your toes gripping the floor. Your feet should be wider than shoulder width apart and your knees bent, as if in a wide squat position (or as if you were riding on horseback). Keep your back straight and turn your upper body to the side, looking in the direction of the attack. Raise your fist to guard position. Turn your back foot in to a 45-degree angle away from the direction of the attack and shift your body weight so that it is supported by your back leg. Pull the knee of the front leg up toward the chest as far as possible. Keep your heel close to the leg as you pull up. Keep your toes back as far as possible. You will be kicking with the heel of that foot. Rotate the upper body and hips away from the direction of the kick while thrusting the kicking leg out directly to the side at your target. Immediately retract your kicking leg following the strike and return to your original position.

THE LOWDOWN

HIP LOVE

Love your hips. Use them to your advantage. Use their power to add force to your strike.

If you've never taken this type of class or done any martial arts in the past, you should definitely take the time to be an observer first. If you see that the instructor is advocating lightning speed repetitions with no regard to form, look out. You may end up pulling a muscle or injuring a joint or two.

As with most group fitness classes, cut yourself some slack. It will take a little bit of time to get used to kickboxing techniques. Ancient Asian warriors went through several years of disciplined training in order to perfect their life-preserving art. Don't be disappointed if you aren't stunningly successful right away.

Cardio kickboxing is generally an equipment-free class. Dress in something that will be comfortable and allow for free movement. Often this class is taught barefoot. It is a nice feeling to be able to let your feet feel the ground beneath them. If you are not comfortable with foot exposure, it is also fine to keep your shoes on. Any type of training shoe will work, but a cross-training shoe is recommended for extra support. Make sure to bring a towel and water.

DANCE

Going into a class as a new student, while the rest of the class has been rehearsing a combination for weeks, can be quite discouraging and disappointing. This is the thing to remember: If you're entering a class as a novice in the middle of a program where everyone else has been practicing the moves for weeks, you *will* be lost. You may be able to pick up the moves very easily, but if you have no dance experience, chances are you won't. Trust us when we tell you that you are not the problem. This is absolutely normal. If you aren't worried about getting all the steps and just want to enjoy yourself, go for it. If you're worried about feeling like the ugly duckling in a lake of graceful and coordinated swans, here is our advice: Talk to the instructor before class and ask where the class is in a routine. Is it the

first week? Have they been working on a routine for many weeks? If it is the first or maybe even the second week, try the class. Try it, and stick with it. You'll see yourself progress as the weeks go on and you will begin to feel a peculiar feeling of nostalgia for the Solid Gold Dancers (or perhaps the Fly Girls).

THE LOWDOWN
PRIVATE DANCER

The thought of taking a dance class has always terrified you, although, when Jennifer Lopez's latest music video comes on TV, you push the coffee table out of the way and bust a move, pretending you're one of her backup dancers. You're reluctant to get your groove on in public, but in the privacy of your bedroom, you've mastered all the moves in *Footloose* and *Flash Dance*. Does this sound like you? Well if does, we recommend that you sign up for a dance class immediately, even if you're afraid to. Share yourself with the world and have fun while you are doing it. Dance classes are a great way to get over your inhibitions.

GROUP FITNESS CLASSES

The great thing about dance classes is that there are so many different types to choose from. One of them is bound to tickle your fancy. They're all meant to be fun and will give you a good cardio work-out in the meantime. Below we have listed some dance classes you'll find out there. This list is certainly not all-encompassing. It is merely here to give you an idea of the vastness of your options when it comes to dance.

- African Dance
- Ballet and ballet-related classes such as Ballet Barre class
- Ballroom Dancing
- Belly Dancing
- Broadway Dancing
- Cha-Cha
- Funk
- Hip Hop
- Jazz
- Mambo
- Merengue
- Salsa
- Samba
- Striptease
- Tango
- Two-Stepping

There is no specific dress requirement for dance classes, and depending on the type of dance, you may or may not be wearing any shoes. Be an observer of the class before you become a participant and take note of what others in the class are wearing. Your best bet would be to follow their general guidelines.

Give yourself a chance to get down and boogie. You may even be surprised at how good you are!

GLIDING

Gliding is a group fitness aerobics class that uses sliding discs.

WHY GLIDE?

Gliding will strengthen your heart, improve your sense of balance and stability, and help you develop graceful, fluid movement. It's a fun, a low-impact workout that anyone can do.

THE CHRONICLES

The gliding program was created by a very well-known and experienced fitness instructor, Mindy Mylrea. She was named International Instructor of the Year in 1999/2000, is a former National and World Aerobic Champion and is one of the most enthusiastic and fun instructors we know. Mindy is accomplished in many areas of fitness and is the star of a plethora of fitness videos. You can learn more about her on her Web site, www.jumpincfitness.com.

THE INSIGHT

Gliding is a simple, yet ingenious concept. The equipment is basically a pair of nine-inch, super-lightweight purple plastic sliding discs. These discs are used on the floor and propelled through the movements with your feet or hands, depending on the exercise. The idea, like other equipment depriving you of the certainty of a steady floor, is to force your body to engage the core and other stabilizing muscles throughout the range of motion. Working with the discs will help you to improve your sense of balance and increase your core strength. The noteworthy and unique quality of these playful purple saucers, setting them apart from most other destabilizing equipment out there, is that while you are able to work both sides of the body simultaneously, each side also operates independently of the other. Your brain is assigned the extra duty of quickly reacting to each unsteady side separately but at the same time. Practice with the glide system will help even the clumsiest of us to move like charming and graceful ballerinas.

GROUP FITNESS CLASSES

Fundamental to gliding success is foot positioning. For most exercises done in the standing position, place the balls of your feet directly in the center of the discs, with the heels of your feet extended off the back edge. This position will give you the most stability and control because it allows you to use your heel as a brake. Should you feel yourself losing control, you'll be able to easily stop the movement and regain composure by simply shifting your weight back onto the floor. For most exercises done from either a seated or a lying position on the floor, keep your feet flexed and place the heels of your feet in the center of the discs with the balls of the feet hanging off the front edge. Some exercises invoke the use of your hands instead of your feet. The positioning of your hands will vary from exercise to exercise.

For the most control, keep most of your weight centered over the nonsliding foot and your heel down in "brake" position. As a beginner, Mindy suggests trying exercises that involve single-disc gliding only, with one foot on the floor and the other on the saucer, until you get a feel for the sliding movement. When you begin to have better command of the movement, try double-disc gliding exercises with one saucer under each foot.

The glide system was developed to function as a class on its own, and as an addition to almost any other type of class. For example, you may find a Glide-Yoga class, a Glide-Step class, or a Glide-Conditioning class at your gym. In a full Gliding class, the moves through the duration of the class will be cardio-focused, strength-focused, or some sort of combination of the two.

If your gym offers a Gliding class, it will have invested in gliders for you to use. Depending on the focus of the class you're taking, the gliding discs may or may not be the only piece of equipment necessary for class. Confer with your instructor beforehand to be sure. In any case, the gym should provide any other equipment you may be using. Though you'll practice moving with the fluidity and flow of a ballerina, here is a word to the wise: Gliders, gracefully refuse your inner child's desire to wear a tutu to class. It will take away, not add to, your charm. Snug-fitting and comfortable workout attire will work best. Regarding foot dress, pointe shoes are also not recommended. A supportive aerobic or cross-training shoe is recommended for extra reinforcement during lateral movements. Bring a towel and water, please.

GYROTONICS

Training based on the gyrotonic expansion system of strengthening and stretching in a circular motion.

WHY GYROTONICS?

Gyrotonics is a nonimpact form of exercise that will tone your muscles and increase strength, flexibility, and range of motion.

THE CHRONICLES

Gyrotonics was introduced to the United States in the 1980s and developed by a man named Juiliu Horvath using the fundamental ideologies of yoga, gymnastics, ballet, and swimming. The movements are designed to integrate multijoint motions and to therapeutically increase range of motion, flexibility, alignment, coordination, and core strength.

THE INSIGHT

Gyrotonic stems from the root *gyro*, a Greek word that means "ring" or "spiral"; a *tonic* is something that serves to stimulate or energize. The gyrotonic expansion system, in short, is based on pulleys that will allow several variations of circular motions with resistance. The system is used to strengthen and stretch muscles and connective tissues surrounding the joints of the body.

Although gyrotonics is becoming increasingly popular, you're not likely to find the gyrotonic expansion system in most gyms. It is usually available in private studios, often associated with rehabilitation, dance, and Pilates, and must be taught by a specially certified gyrotonics trainer. A gyrotonics studio will have several pieces of equipment specific to the practice, and appropriate dress falls within the same boundaries as that of a Yoga or Pilates class. Clothing should be flexible but form-fitting, in order to allow your instructor to see and correct your form if necessary. You will be barefoot while doing gyrotonics.

> Gyrokinesis is the group fitness version of gyrotonics. The philosophy within the movements of gyrokinesis is the same as that of gyrotonics, but without the equipment.

HEAVY HOOP CLASS

A class surrounding the use of a large weighted ring, similar to a heavy Hula Hoop.

WHY HEAVY HOOP?

Heavy Hoop class will strengthen your heart and provide a great way to increase muscle strength and endurance. Some say it can also help create a muscularly balanced body. It's a low-impact workout suitable for anyone. It is also very enjoyable and may trigger some happy Hula Hooping memories.

THE CHRONICLES

The Heavy Hoop is a weighted Hula Hoop developed by Wendy Iverson, an aerobics instructor and personal trainer, initially, as a way for women to work off post-baby weight. Its original version was a good old-fashioned Hula Hoop, stuffed with a telephone wire, padded with piping insulation, and duct-taped together. It has come a long way since then, and is now a metal ring covered with high-quality foam. It is available in a three-pound version for a beginner workout, as well as a five-pound version for a more advanced Heavy Hooping workout. The Heavy Hoop class is a fairly recent notion, first introduced into fitness in 2002.

THE INSIGHT

The Heavy Hoop can be used as a cardiovascular tool for a fun-filled, low-impact workout or as a resistance-training tool capable of working all of your major muscle groups. Some instructors may keep you Heavy Hooping in some capacity for the entire time, while others may complement the workout with auxiliary equipment. Refer to the instructor for a class prelude and guidance.

Dress for "Hoops" as you would any other aerobics class, in comfortably close-fitting clothing. Keep in mind that midriff-baring tops may not be such a good choice for this type of workout as the skin around your waistline will not appreciate the continuous assault of the hoop. Definitely wear laterally supportive footwear such as cross-training shoes, and bring your towel and water. Although we haven't actually tried this novel exercise, we feel it's our duty to give you the option to explore it.

INDOOR CYCLING (SPINNING)

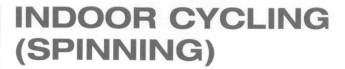

Indoor cycling is a group fitness training experience on stationary bikes.

WHY SPIN?

Indoor cycling is a low-impact workout that strengthens your heart and is gentle on the joints. You can do this activity for long periods of time and through to your golden years without causing stress to the knee and hip joints. It's a great way to lower your body fat percentage and increase your overall fitness level. The combined simplicity and rhythmic flow of the class create a great template for practicing the mind-body connection.

THE CHRONICLES

The indoor cycling phenomenon began in the late 1980s in California. It has since increased in popularity and can be found on group fitness schedules in gyms around the world. It is a class that appeals to many different types of people, from the passionate, competitive cyclist training for an upcoming race season to the newest gym member who's never worked out and hasn't been on a bicycle in years. Indoor cycling is one of the most easily adaptable training mediums offered at gyms. It caters to all, from the well-seasoned athlete to the less-than-conditioned fitness newbie.

THE LOWDOWN

CYCLING FORMATS

Indoor Cycling classes may vary in format and focus; you may encounter some of the following:

Endurance ride—This class is formulated to take your heart rate up to a certain zone and maintain it in that range for the majority of the class.

Interval ride—This is a very popular type of class that can be broken down into two groups——short, super demanding intervals followed by longer periods of recovery, and longer, not quite as intense intervals followed by shorter or equal periods of recovery. Classes may incorporate a combination of both approaches.

THE INSIGHT

Veteran cyclists and ardent fans who have taken spinning classes for a very long time may make it seem cultlike in nature. Most have their own butt-hugging padded shorts and slick cycling shoes, and you may notice some avid cyclists checking their heart rate monitors incessantly. When you peek into an Indoor Cycling class, the flurry of intense, fast-moving legs, the loud music, and the dark, vaultlike nature of the studio may send you running off in the opposite direction. As you quickly retreat to a safer part of the gym, you may be wondering: Am I in good enough shape to take this class? How do I set up that kind of bike? Do I need a heart rate monitor? Do I need special shoes to take the class? Do I have to wear those cycling shorts? Maybe that class is only for experienced cyclists and not for novices like me.

Here are the answers to those questions: No, you don't have to be in any particular shape to take an Indoor Cycling class. You are always in full control of the speed of your legs and how much resistance you have on the bike. The intensity of your ride is always relative to your personal level of conditioning and your fitness program, and is revealed to outsiders at your sole

discretion. You never have to feel like you are competing with your classmates because you are the only one who knows exactly what your intensity is. There is really no choreography involved with Indoor Cycling classes, so any concerns that you will be twirling in the wrong direction and stepping on your neighbor's toes can be instantly dismissed. Cycling shorts, shoes, and a heart rate monitor are always optional. It is a great class for all levels, especially beginners, for these reasons.

With this class, it's particularly important to arrive 10 to 15 minutes early, proclaim your inexperience to the instructor, and ask questions.

- **How do I set up my bike?**
- **Can you give me any pointers on technique?**
- **Is there anything I should know about how you lead your class?**
- **How will I know what intensities to ride?**
- **This is also a good time to expose any conditions that may be cause for modifying the workout such as being pregnant or recovering from injury.**

105

A heart rate monitor is certainly not necessary for taking this class, but is a very useful tool. It will help keep you focused, provide you with objective feedback, and teach you about your body. (Polar makes very good ones. Check out www.polarusa.com.) Regarding foot gear, a training shoe with a stiffer sole is a way to go. Over time, if you develop a strong affinity for this class, you may want to consider investing in a pair of cycling shoes—once you experience how smooth a ride in them feels, you may never want to ride in ordinary sneakers again. In truth, the bike seat is not particularly comfortable, especially in the beginning. A good antidote for this discomfort is a padded seat (or a gel seat). You can usually buy one from your gym. Ask at the front desk or the gym store. Cycling shorts are another very soothing alternative. You can pick up a pair at any cycling shop. Regarding attire, trade in your big, baggy sweatpants for lighter, less cumbersome shorts. They will keep you cooler and are less likely to get caught on the moving parts of the bike during your ride. Bring a towel to dry off and water or some type of sports drink to keep hydrated.

THE LOWDOWN

IT'S NOT THE TOUR DE FRANCE
Don't worry about keeping up with everyone else around you. The main goal for your first few classes is to make it through from start to finish.

BIKE SETUP

Bike setup is one of the most important things to know when taking a Spinning class. Proper setup can make your ride so much more comfortable and effective.

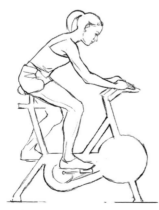

THIS IS WHAT YOU SHOULD LOOK LIKE WHEN PROPERLY SET UP ON YOUR BIKE.

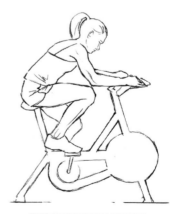

THIS IS WHAT YOU SHOULD *NOT* LOOK LIKE.

Always have enough resistance to support your body weight with your legs when riding out of the saddle. Your body should not move uncontrollably at any point. Keep in mind that riding out of the saddle is always optional. Ride in the saddle until you feel experienced enough to stand.

Be sure to keep your knees aligned with your hips throughout your pedal stroke. Do not let your knees jut out to the sides or nearly bang into each other. When setting yourself up on the bike, here are a few posture pointers you will relentlessly need to remind yourself of, especially during the first few months of indoor cycling. You may want to write them down and keep them somewhere visible, perhaps on the handlebars in front of you, until they become an embedded habit.

- Hinge forward at the hips.
- Tilt the pelvis back slightly.
- Bring the heels of your hands to the handlebars with your fingers (including your thumbs) up and over the handlebars.
- Relax your grip.
- Unlock your elbows.
- Drop your shoulders.
- Keep your chin off your chest with your focus out in front of you.
- Allow your back to be softly rounded.

THE LOWDOWN
RAW RUMP

As a novice indoor cyclist, you may feel assaulted by the narrow and barely cushioned bike seat, especially if you're seated for extended periods of time. Consider purchasing a gel seat or cycling shorts, or both for that matter. We guarantee that they will help tremendously, and please don't let this potential source of discomfort deter you from taking a cycling class. Strangely enough, your body will adapt——you'll get used to the feeling of your weight on your rear end on that itty-bitty seat. If you feel like you really need to stand to relieve your discomfort, ride a stint out of the saddle. Be sure to have enough resistance to carry your weight before doing it. You'll know that you need to add resistance if, when you stand, you feel you are running through air and are dropping quickly through the top of each pedal stroke. Ask your instructor to give you pointers on riding out of the saddle.

JUMP ROPE CLASS

This group fitness class embraces the fundamental techniques of jumping rope for fire-charged cardiovascular aerobic and anaerobic training.

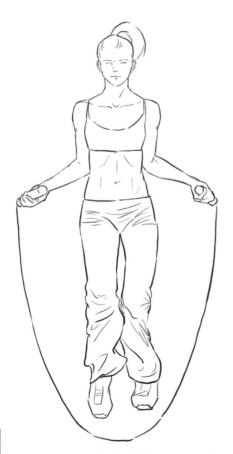

WHY JUMP ROPE?

Jumping rope is a marvelous aerobic and anaerobic total body workout. It tones the muscles and will help improve speed, agility, power, coordination, and balance.

THE CHRONICLES

Jumping rope, sometimes called rope skipping, is actually a competitive sport. It was developed as such by Richard Cendali, a physical education instructor, in the 1980s. In group fitness, it has long been a part of youth programs and made its way into gyms as an offspring of boxing classes.

THE LOWDOWN

THE HEAVY

For an extra jump rope challenge, use a heavy rope. Such ropes are evenly weighted and available in two- three- five- and eight-pound varieties. Don't be mistaken; even the two-pound rope makes for an incredibly challenging workout. (To purchase a heavy rope, see www.performbetter.com.)

JUMPING ROPE

GROUP FITNESS CLASSES

THE INSIGHT

Jump Rope classes will come in assorted varieties. Some classes will not diverge from their titles and be nothing but choreographed rope skipping. Others will infuse a variety of different body sculpting elements into the class and use the jump rope segments as intense cardio burst intervals. These classes, especially at the intermediate and advanced levels, are generally pretty fast-paced. For a beginner, even the introductory classes may seem fast. Don't be discouraged. Do your best and stick with it. A little practice will get you moving as quickly as anyone else in the class. Regarding technique, here are some tips to help you get the most out of your jumping time.

- Roll your shoulders down and into your back. They should feel relaxed.

- Do not let your elbows flair out to the sides. Keep them close to your body.

- Keep your wrists slightly below your elbows.

- Use your wrists to turn the rope, not your arms and shoulders.

- Land softly. Keep your knees very soft to absorb the landing.

- Jump from the balls of your feet and land on the balls of your feet.

- Don't think of it as jumping up, but rather just barely letting the rope slip under your feet.

- Let the rope travel around you in a tight, high arc. There should be no slack in the rope.

- Avoid whipping your neighbor with your rope and be sure to have ample room around you in class.

The ropes used in Jump Rope class will not be the ones you double-dutched with as a kid, and your gym will set you up with whatever type of rope you need. Wearing super-baggy clothing to this class may not be the best choice. Self-lassoing tricks caused by excess fabric can be dangerous and humbling, though are likely to amuse the casual observer. We recommend sticking to comfortable, flexible, and breathable clothing you can move freely in but wouldn't be tangled in. You don't need any type of special training shoes for Jump Rope classes, although we recommend a cross-training shoe that will support lateral movements.

MIND/BODY INTEGRATED TRAINING CLASS

The concept of the mind being directly connected to and influencing the capabilities of the body is at the forefront of the fitness world. Ancient civilizations knew this long before we did. Although we often hear stories of people overcoming astoundingly dismal circumstances and beating the odds in the face of seeming impossibility, we aren't usually able to personally identify with this ability. We have somehow ignored this connection for a long time and only now are beginning to re-acknowledge and accentuate the crucial significance of mind over matter, or better stated, matter by means of mind. How we perceive our body affects how our body reacts. The mind says stop; the body stops. The body surges forward with fierce determination when the mind believes it can. This is a prominent approach to fitness that is still developing. It is a mind-set that can be integrated into any class you take, and on a grander scale, into anything you do in life.

There are a few classes, besides Yoga and Pilates, worth mentioning that truly flourish in this area. One you may have heard of is Tai Chi. It is an active meditation derived from Taoism, and is designed to harmonize the body, mind, and emotions. Tai Chi's origins can be traced back to China nearly 1,000 years ago. Some others are IntenSati and Will Power & Grace. Check out their Web sites: www.intensati.com and www.willpower productions.info. You will find that these classes, aside from the practice of weaving together the mind and body, will also provide a substantial workout. Depending on the class, in many instances you will also get a fierce and invigorating cardiovascular, strength-building, core and flexibility training.

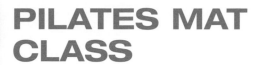

PILATES MAT CLASS

Pilates is a methodical practice of very specific exercises and focused breathing patterns meant to work the whole body as well as the mind.

WHY PILATES?

Pilates will increase strength and flexibility while toning the muscles and is an especially effective way to strengthen your body's core muscles.

THE CHRONICLES

It is difficult to talk about Pilates, the work, without mentioning Pilates, the man. So here's a little bit of history.

Joseph Pilates, born in Germany in 1880, was an unhealthy child who suffered from asthma, rickets, and rheumatoid fever. In an attempt to improve his strength and overall health, he studied anatomy and various forms of exercise. Eventually conquering his ailments, Pilates became an avid sportsman, and he was known to box, dive, ski, and practice gymnastics.

During the First World War, Pilates was forced into internment in the United Kingdom, and it was there that he developed his method of rehabilitation. He used the springs in the beds as resistance equipment and combined that with methods of breathing.

Pilates immigrated to the United States and, along with his wife Clara, opened up a gym in New York City in 1926 using the concept he developed during his internment in the United Kingdom. The gym was located near many dance schools and soon became extremely popular in dance circles. Pilates' amazing work was hugely beneficial in helping dancers recover from injury. His method of exercise and rehabilitation has reached far beyond the circles of dance and is currently practiced throughout the world. Joseph Pilates taught in his studio until he died in 1967 at the age of 87.

THE INSIGHT

The equipment used in Pilates today is based on the original bedspring concept. The idea is to exercise using nonimpact resistance, so that there is no stress to the joints. Some pieces of equipment you may encounter are the Cadillac, Reformer, Chair, and Barrel.

With that being said, in most traditional gyms, you will not find this type of equipment. The majority of classes you will encounter are mat based. Do not be discouraged or turned off by this. Mat classes are a great way to experience Pilates at all levels, but especially as a beginner. This "smart" body work will help you grow stronger, become more flexible, especially in the abdominals and back muscles, and help correct your alignment. It will help you become more mentally and physically coordinated, and will improve your posture, core strength, and

body awareness. You will also experience an increase in balance and control of your body.

So, what exactly will you be doing in a Pilates mat class? you may be wondering. We are getting to that. Pilates mat classes are a series of floor exercises designed to align and strengthen your body from your foundation, or your core. There are 500 different exercises based on six specific ideas—centering, concentration, control, precision, breathing, and flowing movement. We apologize, but we won't be providing details on all 500 exercises. For that, you'll need to get a book that is all about Pilates. What we have provided instead are a few basic Pilates mat exercises, very rudimentary descriptions of what they are, and their benefits. This should help give you an idea of what the exercises are about.

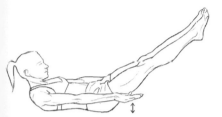

THE ONE HUNDREDS

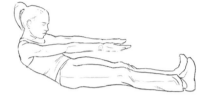

ROLL-UP

The one hundreds—This is definitely one of the most well-known Pilates exercises. Perform one hundred specialized sit-ups. Your arms and legs remain straight and off the ground, and your abdominals remain contracted the whole time. Flutter your arms up and down, as if you were pumping them and focus on exhaling forcefully. This will teach you how to stabilize the pelvis and strengthen the abdominals. It will also get your blood moving and increase circulation.

Roll-up—Roll up your body from a lying position into a seated one very slowly. This focuses on the spine.

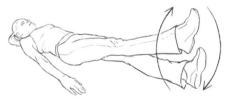

LEG CIRCLES

Leg circles—Lying flat on your back, make controlled circles with one leg while keeping the rest of your body in a steady position flat on the floor. This will boost movement in your hip joints and strengthen the inner thighs, pelvis, and stabilizers.

ROLLING LIKE A BALL

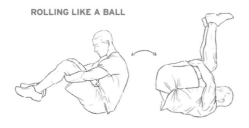

Rolling like a ball—Curl your body in a ball and roll back and forth. This will stretch and activate the spine. You will also be focusing on engaging your abdominal muscles.

SINGLE-LEG STRETCH

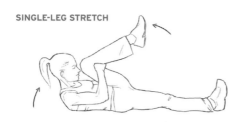

Single-leg stretch—Lying flat on the ground, bring one knee in and curl your head and shoulders off the ground so that your forehead meets that knee. Keep the other leg extended and on the ground in front of you. This will increase the movement of the hips and knees and strengthen the abdominals.

SPINE STRETCH

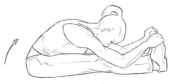

Spine stretch—From a seated position with your legs and back straight, curl your torso and reach for your toes. This will stretch your hamstrings and spine.

THE SAW

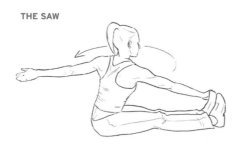

Saw—From a seated position with your legs and back straight and your arms out to the sides, twist and curl your torso so that your hand reaches for the opposite foot. This will improve your ability to rotate the torso and will teach you how to stabilize your hips.

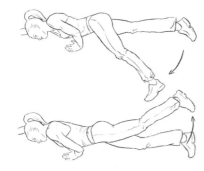

SIDE KICKS

Side kicks—Lying on one side with your body aligned from head to toe, reach your top leg forward and back. Your leg should be straight and parallel to the ground, and your hips and upper body stable throughout the movement.

Seal—From a seated position with your knees bent and out to the sides, wrap your hands around the heels of your feet. Curl your spine and lift your knees so that you are balancing on your sit bones. Roll back, lifting your hips as far off the ground as you can. Roll back up to starting position, balanced on your sit bones. This will stretch your spine and work on balance and control.

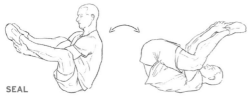

SEAL

In a Pilates mat class, you may find that the only tool required is the mat itself. Others may make use of medicine balls, Physio Balls, or a Pilates "Magic Ring" (a springy metal ring). They are each used to do various toning exercises targeting specific muscles. No need to run out to your neighborhood Pilates supply shop; your gym will provide you with any equipment called for in the particular class you are taking. Your Pilates outfit should resemble that of your Yoga class. It should be flexible, but form-fitting, in order to allow your instructor to see and correct your form if necessary. Naked toes will command the Pilates floor, so clean feet are a must. Keep externally dry and internally hydrated with your ever-essential towel and water.

STRETCH CLASS

Stretch classes are designed to guide the participants to increased flexibility.

WHY STRETCH?

Stretching provides both physical and mental relaxation and will help reduce muscle soreness and tension. You'll learn safe and effective ways of stretching while also enhancing muscle awareness and improving your flexibility.

THE INSIGHT

What's to it? Everyone knows how to stretch, even your kitty cat, right? Wrong. Think again. That you reach your arms and legs out toward the bedposts when you wake up is great, and may help get you out of bed. But if you want to reap the full benefits of stretching, you're going to have to do a bit more than that. The idea of a class on stretching may seem like time poorly spent at the gym. In actuality, stretching is a very well-studied practice and there is extensively documented rhyme and reason for doing it. But be careful; if you don't perform your stretches carefully and skillfully, you can cause damage to your body.

If you are new to stretching, and are looking to improve your flexibility, or if you have some experience and an avid interest in delving deeper, consider taking a Stretch class. This type of class, which normally lasts for 15 to 45 minutes, will teach you how to stretch safely and effectively. It's difficult to describe exactly what you'll be doing in a specific Stretch class because there are so many different schools of stretching—isometric stretching, active isolated stretching, static and dynamic stretching—and each form is valid for a host of reasons. The direction of the class is determined by the instructor. Some classes will incorporate the use of stretching tools such as straps and bands, while others will be constructed around nothing more than the use of your body. You may also find Pilates- or yoga-based stretches integrated into a class. Have a conversation with the instructor whose class you're considering to get a beat on exactly what type of stretching the class will be doing. Let them know you are new to the class and have them help you through the moves so that you are able to get the most out of the session.

TREADMILL CLASS

Although Treadmill classes may go by many names, the nature of such classes is pretty straightforward. You use a treadmill and manipulate your speed and level of incline in a structured class led by an instructor.

WHY TREADMILL CLASS?

Running will strengthen your heart. A Treadmill class will teach you how to make your running more interesting and effective. It's a great way to learn new techniques and strategies for running on your own both indoors and outdoors.

THE INSIGHT

Ever find yourself on a treadmill running haphazardly with no real focus? If you enjoy high-intensity walking, jogging, or running, whether indoors or outdoors, and are looking for a way to do it with more decided rhyme or reason or are perhaps seeking a way to train for an event, you may have plenty to gain from taking a treadmill class. Without experience or guidance, it is difficult to devise a plan that will help you progress in a safe and sensible way. Treadmill classes are generally led by instructors who are trained runners themselves. The instructor will guide you through a 20- to 60-minute program. He or she will ask you to utilize different speeds and ramp inclines to simulate varying terrains with the greater goal of developing a combination of speed, endurance, and efficiency.

Many times, Treadmill classes are taught in intervals, mixing running with another mode of cardiovascular training such as cycling on a stationary bike, resistance, or core training. Check your class schedule for the exact description of the format of the class you're considering.

For all women, a good, supportive sports bra is essential when running. It will minimize uncomfortable bouncing and possible "falling out." For all men, compression shorts are a must for the same reasons. This is the time to bust out the running shoes. They will provide the most cushioning and will minimize the impact on your joints.

URBAN REBOUNDING

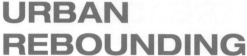

Urban Rebounding is an exhilarating and unique cardiovascular-focused class taught on mini-trampolines, also known as rebounders.

WHY URBAN REBOUND?

This class will strengthen your heart. The soft surface of the rebounder absorbs the shock that would normally be felt on the joints, making this class a low-impact workout that in fact has a strengthening and stabilizing effect. It is appropriate for all ages and will increase your coordination and balance and increase your over-all fitness level. The rebounder allows you to work at a relatively high intensity for a longer period of time with surprising ease and comfort, and because it bears such an unusual resemblance to the once forbidden act of bouncing on your parents' mattress, it satisfies a devilish childhood desire for mischief.

THE CHRONICLES

Rebounders have been part of the fitness world since the 1960s and were introduced into group fitness by a good friend of ours, J. B. Burns, in New York City in the late 1990s. His passion for rebounding blossomed from a knee injury. In search of a workout that would be intense and thorough, and simultaneously gentle on his recovering knee, he developed the Urban Rebounding class. The class is choreographed using basic old-school high-low moves to music. The traditional Urban Rebounding class includes a cardio segment, a set of sport-specific intervals, and a simple body conditioning segment of squats, push-ups, and triceps dips, and ends with core work. You will also find a variety of other formats that may have a stronger emphasis on sports-specific training, dance, plyometric, or body conditioning moves than the traditional class format. Check your class schedule for the specific details.

GROUP FITNESS CLASSES

THE INSIGHT

Don't worry; no back flips or circus tricks necessary. The biggest fears surrounding this class involve thoughts of falling or bouncing off the rebounder, breaking through the mat of the rebounder, or not being coordinated enough to follow the choreography.

Contrary to logic, there is essentially no jumping involved. Reverse your thinking. When on the rebounder, you should always focus on pushing down, as if trying to punch through the mat with the balls of your feet. The mat is strong enough to hold up to 300 pounds, so chances are you're not going to be able to actually punch a hole through it. The moves are made to be uncomplicated and easy to follow. During your first few classes you'll go through a natural period of adjustment, and we admit, it will feel a bit awkward. This is normal, and everyone goes through it. The good news is that the learning curve is quick for most and you

do not need to perform the moves perfectly in order to get the benefits of the class. Don't give up and abandon the class just because you feel like you're not getting it. Chances are you are only a few bounces away from catching up.

Get to class a few minutes early and ask the instructor for a quick demonstration of the fundamental moves. Choose cross-trainers over running sneakers for this particular type of class. They provide much more lateral support. Sweatpants or any other wide-bottomed long pants are not recommended for this class. Precarious moments may arise from the loose material getting caught on the spring's midbounce. Be sure to bring a towel to class, not only to wipe off your sweat, but also to prevent your hair from getting caught on the springs of the rebounder during the core segment.

YOGA

A class that simultaneously exercises the mind, body, and spirit through postures and breathing techniques, and is derived from ancient eastern teachings.

WHY YOGA?

Yoga will increase strength and flexibility and tone your muscles while also increasing peace of mind, balance, and stability and your ability to focus. Physical, mental, and emotional stress can be relieved, and contrary to popular reservations about beginning a yoga practice, there are no prerequisites (like super flexibility or spiritual inclinations) required to begin. Anyone can do it.

THE CHRONICLES

The history of yoga can be traced back over 5,000 years and is believed to have grown out of shamanism of the Stone Age. Relative to this, it is still extremely new to the western world. It has gained a huge amount of attention and popularity in the past 30 to 40 years. Essentially, yoga is an extensive collection of spiritual practices designed to integrate the mind, body, and spirit. There are many different styles of yoga and while they may vary in approach, they share this ultimate goal.

THE LOWDOWN

THE MEANING OF YOGA
The word *yoga* originates from the Sanskrit root *yui*, which means "to yoke" or "to join together."

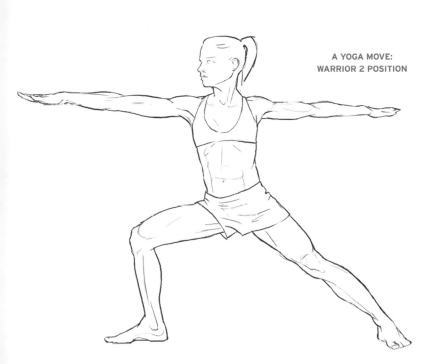

A YOGA MOVE:
WARRIOR 2 POSITION

THE FRINGE BENEFITS OF A YOGA PRACTICE

RELAXATION—The stretches and breathing techniques used in yoga help release tension and can help calm the nervous system.

CONCENTRATION AND FOCUS—Practicing balancing postures in yoga will foster body awareness. This, along with mindful movement, will help build concentration and focus.

TONING—Yoga postures are, in essence, isometric exercises and will tone your muscles.

FLEXIBILITY—Yoga will delicately stretch your muscles, allowing you to become more flexible.

121

THE INSIGHT

No, yoga is not a religion, and no, you do not need to go through any ritualistic ceremonies in order to practice it. Seeing people twisted up in unconventional positions and chanting in foreign languages may lead some people to think so. Many people shy away from trying yoga because it is so completely different from anything else going on in a gym. The instructors are not asking students for the common push-up and jumping jack. Instead they're giving verbal cues that would implicate the imitation of some type of dangerous reptile (cobra) or some game your Jack Russell terrier likes to play (Upward Facing Dog, Downward Facing Dog, Corpse Pose). The regulars in the class can bend forward, backward, sideways, and through any given uncommon direction with ease and grace. Do you remember when you were a child and you had the ability to bend and stretch every which way without a thought? You didn't worry about tweaking your back when tumbling around with your brothers and sisters, or simply even reaching down and touching your toes. Well, yoga will allow your body to rediscover the flexibility it had in its youthful years. In addition, your body will become stronger and more fluid. It won't happen immediately. Getting the hang of holding your body in positions it's not accustomed to being in will take some time. Becoming good at yoga will require a certain amount of dedication and commitment, as with anything you'd like to become good at. People who have been practicing yoga for a long time and are able to assume the contorted,

pretzel like poses were probably not always as flexible as they are now.

A peculiarity of some yoga classes is the chanting that goes on. You may not feel comfortable "ohm"ing and "aah"ing in public. This is normal. As Westerners, most of us are not used to public group incantations (what goes on privately is another story). Chanting is not a necessary part of doing yoga, but it certainly makes the experience a bit more authentic. The chants in yoga have historic and spiritual significance. They are also a great form of release and foster a sense of kinship in the class. Try it. It can be weird, but in a wonderful sort of way.

Yoga classes can be longer in duration than most group fitness classes. They are typically about an hour to two hours long. This may seem like too much of a commitment for someone who may merely desire yogic experimentation. There isn't much we can say about this. Just do it. Commit to it and don't think about it. The time will fly by.

Given the many different types of yoga, figuring out which style is right for you can be somewhat overwhelming. To give you an idea we briefly describe a few below. In the United States, most Yoga classes are based on Hatha yoga. Literally, *Hatha* means "sun" and "moon." It aims to integrate the body and spirit through several yoga postures, or "asanas," and yoga breathing, or "pranayama." Most modern yoga does not emphasize the esoteric yogic foundation; instead, it focuses on the postures and breathing aspect.

TYPES OF YOGA

As a beginner, try yoga styles that focus on alignment such as Hatha, Iyengar, and Kripalu.

Hatha yoga—This is a less-demanding and gentle method of yoga. Its main focus is on alignment and posture, overall strength, flexibility, and breath.

Ashtanga or power yoga—Ashtanga is made up of a rigid sequence of postures. It emphasizes continuous fast-paced movement with synchronized breathing throughout the practice. Power yoga is a spin-off of Ashtanga, making use of postures that are more creative in progression. Both are athletic practices. We would not recommend either class for first-time yoga dabblers.

Bikram or hot yoga—This is a strict series of 26 poses that are performed in a room heated to 100 degrees Fahrenheit and higher. You will definitely be sweating throughout this experience. (Do not plan to go out on a date without a shower after this class.) The idea is that by keeping your muscles warm, you will be able to achieve greater flexibility. This intense heat will also foster greater mental endurance. In order to stay hydrated throughout this class, where you will be losing water through sweat from the heat, arrive already hydrated. You may be asked to refrain from drinking water until the specified "drink breaks" in these classes in order to allow for an undistracted flow from posture to posture. If you are feeling dehydrated and need to drink outside of the scheduled water breaks, respectfully do so—the side effects of dehydration can be quite serious.

Iyengar—This form of yoga focuses on the technical aspect of each pose, emphasizing its therapeutic benefits. A lot of attention is placed on alignment and props are heavily used. Iyengar is a great form of yoga for beginners.

Kripalu—Gentle and spiritually focused, Kripalu is also a good choice for beginners. It is a three-stage approach where inner focus and meditation are incorporated within the yoga poses.

Kundalini—This is a vigorous, stimulating, and esoteric style of yoga. It mixes breathing techniques, movement, poses, and chanting with the intention of conjuring up the inactive spiritual energy at the base of the spine.

Sivananda—This approach to yoga is traditional with a rigid structure of advanced poses, breathing, and meditation. Not really a great starting place for beginners.

MOMMY YOGA

Many yoga studios offer yoga classes that are specifically designed for pre- and postnatal women. Prenatal yoga is composed of gentler versions of some of the same yoga postures you would find in a non-baby-related Yoga class. It is tailored to protect moms-to-be and their developing little ones. Innately, yoga and childbearing go hand in hand. An important part of yoga is practicing to link your breath with your postures. This is also an important aspect of giving birth. It will help strengthen a woman's body for childbearing, as well as ease back pain, nausea, and other common pregnancy-related discomforts.

Postnatal Yoga focuses on renewing energy and rebuilding the strength in the core and pelvic muscles lost during pregnancy and child-birth. Depending on the type of birth (vaginal, cesarean, etc.), a new mom can usually begin her postnatal yoga practice somewhere within two and six weeks of giving birth.

Mommy-and-Me classes have also become very popular. The flow from posture to posture in these classes is slow and interactive between the mommy and baby and the focus is on strengthening the bond between the two. Many of the exercises are meant to support the development of the baby's motor skills. The usual age for mommy and baby classes is between four weeks old and crawling.

Please, moms and moms-to-be, do not begin any sort of Prenatal, Postnatal, or Mommy-and-Me class before contacting your doctors and getting their approval!

BREATHING AND YOGA

Although you have been breathing all your life, you haven't quite experienced "breathing" until yoga. Who knew there were so many different ways to breathe? Breathing exercises are a very important part of practicing yoga. Called pranayama, they were developed by ancient yogis for cleansing. Literally, *pranayama* translates to the control or mastery of life force energy. The goal is to be able to cultivate the energy in your body through breath.

This may also translate well in other classes you may take.

THE LOWDOWN
BREATH BASICS

For most pranayama, the breath is slow and steady. With your back straight and your body relaxed, breathe in and out through the nose. Your breath should feel as if it is filling your belly, as opposed to only your chest.

BUILDING STRENGTH IN YOGA

Yoga is a great form of exercise for both toning and strengthening the body, but it will not have the same effects as a "typical" aerobic workout. Unless you are planning to move at lightning speed or with concrete blocks strapped to your limbs and torso, it will not burn as many calories. To help build strength in yoga, practice holding postures for increasingly longer periods of time and look to move on to advanced postures. Ashtanga yoga and power yoga are the cheetahs of yoga, catapulting very quickly from one posture to the next. This will burn more calories and help build strength and stamina.

EQUIPMENT AND CLOTHING FOR YOGA CLASS

The typical tools used in a Yoga class are mats, blocks, and blankets. Most gyms and all yoga studios will provide you with them. The most basic piece of equipment is the yoga mat. If you try yoga and really enjoy it, you may want to purchase your own. The temperature of yoga studios is normally slightly warmer than other classes. This is to help keep your muscles warm and allow you to focus fully on your postures and breathing. Yoga-wear should be loose and flexible but form-fitting. Swathing extra fabric will impede the instructor's view of your body. The instructor needs to be able to see you, in order to make minor corrections to your poses. Think twice about wearing anything that is restrictive around your waist and ankles. The last thing you want to do is to have your attention drift to the tight elastic of your sweatpants digging into your skin. You want to be as unaware as possible of what you are wearing. Jewelry is not recommended, but having a clean, neutral-scented and deodorized body certainly is. You will always be barefoot in this class, so don't forget to also give your feet a good preclass scrubbing. You should bring a towel and water to class as well.

THE LOWDOWN

A LESSON IN SANSKRIT

Sanskrit is one of the oldest known languages. It is the classical language of India, and the language of yoga.

Vinyasa is the flow from one pose into another.

Hatha can literally be broken down into *ha*, meaning "sun," and *tha*, meaning "moon." The practice is about creating harmony within the body.

Asana means posture.

Pranayama can be translated as control or mastery of the breath. In yoga, the breath is used as a means of clearing and cleansing the body and mind.

THE EQUIPMENT

5

JUST as sometimes you can't see the forest for the trees, walking into a gym can seem as foreign and wild as a cold steel jungle. The vast amount of equipment at gyms can give you the feeling of being completely lost without a map. But don't despair; deconstructing this jungle and simply reconfiguring it will arm you with the information you need to approach this new world with confidence and enthusiasm.

Equipment at a gym can be broken down into three main categories: strength training equipment, cardio equipment, and ancillary equipment. You will find that equipment from each category will be grouped together in the same vicinity as others of its own kind. We have broken down this chapter into these categories, providing photographs, descriptions, intended purpose, and benefits of all the equipment. You will notice a sun ☼ beside the pieces of equipment we categorize as "Essential" for the beginner. You will find more in-depth information on how to use what we feel are some of the indispensable or "essential" pieces of equipment in Chapter 6, "The Quick Start." In that chapter we also outline simple training programs making use of this equipment to get you up and training without delay. At this juncture, if you're ready to get started, skip over to Chapter 6 and come back to this chapter when you want to broaden your horizons with other equipment at the gym.

THE LOWDOWN

A GUIDED TOUR

The guides to this steel jungle are all around you. Trainers are there to help you if you have questions about machine setup and technique, so don't be shy about asking. Often you are given a free training session with your gym membership. Use this session as an opportunity to be introduced to some of the gym's equipment. Bear in mind that this will barely scrape the surface. We highly recommend hiring a trainer for a minimum of 10 sessions to help you delve deeper into the world of gym equipment and learn how to use all the apparatus safely and effectively.

STRENGTH TRAINING EQUIPMENT

This area of the gym seems to be the one always provoking the biggest fears. There are many pieces of equipment for each muscle group, each working the muscle from slightly different angles, in slightly different ways. Some equipment affords more guidance throughout the range of motion (machines). Other equipment encourages joint stability (free weights and cables). Think of the equipment like the shoe department of your favorite store. Within the summer shoe selection alone, you will find slippers, sandals, flip-flops, and the like, all with the same basic function, to dress your feet in warm weather. The same goes for the equipment at a gym. It comes in various forms. You'll find strength training machines, as well as free weights and cables. All forms are effective, some giving your body more guidance than others.

Machines are the safest way to begin your tour of the gym. They'll guide your movements from start to finish, and there are no loose parts to drop. The free weights and cables are more advanced and require more focus and skill to use safely. You will be obliged to call upon your muscles' stabilizing skills to move the weight throughout the exercise. With the free weights, you'll also need to be careful not to let them fall. The added stabilizing benefits of working with them, however, will help strengthen the body and prevent future injury more effectively. It is well worth taking the time to familiarize yourself with them. When you become comfortable with the exercises on the machines, modify your workout scheme by substituting free weights and cables for exercises addressing the same muscle groups. Mixing up the types of equipment you work with will keep things interesting. New and exciting moves will keep your body guessing and will continually challenge your fitness level.

THE LOWDOWN

FREE WEIGHTS

The term *free weights* is an umbrella term encompassing dumbbells, bars, and plates.

WEIGHT LOAD

Does your worst recurring nightmare involve the shame and disappointment of investing all your strength and muscle power on a strength training machine without being able to move it because the weight on it is too heavy? You will welcome the return of pleasant dreams and restful slumber when you read this. It is as easy and discreet as inserting the small metal pin into the correct, lighter and more manageable weight plate. The numbers on the plates represent their cumulative weight.

Depending on your free weight of choice, the process of preparing your weight load will sometimes require a greater effort. Dumbbells are as easy as machines to figure out, if not easier (instructions seem ludicrous, but since we are on the subject, here they are). Walk over to the dumbbell rack, select your desired weights, and pick them up. You will find that the racks will be equipped with dumbbells ranging from 5, 8, 10, 12 (or 12.5), 15, sometimes 17 or 17.5, 20, and 25 pounds, and upwards in 5-pound increments until about 100 pounds.

The Olympic bars, however, will require you to load plates on either side. Be sure to load each side evenly and use butterfly clips to secure the plates on the bar in case of an accidental tilting or dropping (you'll see a picture of these things a bit deeper into this chapter). The plates will be available in 2.5, 5, 10, 25, 35, and 45 pounds.

This chapter is organized by body part in the following order: Complete Body, Lower Body, Combo Upper Body, Back, Chest, Shoulders, Biceps, Triceps, and last, but indeed not least, Core.

! **LOOK FOR THE SUN SYMBOL FOR THE ESSENTIAL MACHINES. GET TO KNOW THESE FIRST.**

COMPLETE BODY

☼ SMITH MACHINE

THE FUNCTION This is one of the ultimate strength training machines. It's versatile and can be used independently for a full-body workout. The bar on this machine is track-guided, making all the exercises you do on it safer than its free weight counterparts.

THE EXERCISES Just to give you an idea, you can use this machine to do squats, lunges, bench presses, shoulder presses, and even modified pull-ups. (Voilà, there you have a full-body workout. See page 183 for a full-body "Quick Start" workout using only the Smith machine.) This is not a comprehensive list of all the possible exercises you can do with a Smith machine. That would require a full chapter.

THE BODY PARTS Head to toe

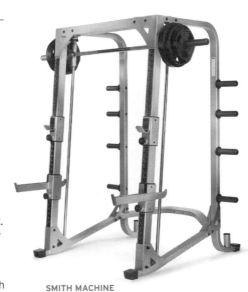

SMITH MACHINE

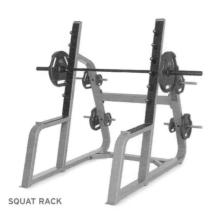

SQUAT RACK

SQUAT RACK

THE FUNCTION This machine is close to a free weight version of the Smith machine and is almost as versatile. As there is no guidance track for the bar, exercises become more challenging.

THE EXERCISES Squats, lunges, dead lifts, bent row, modified pull-ups, shoulder presses, shrugs, biceps curls

THE BODY PARTS Head to toe

CABLES

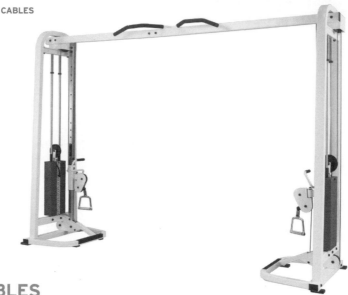

CABLES

We love working out with cables. The things you can do with them number somewhere in the untold thousands. By adjusting the weight and the height setting of the cable, you are able to work just about every muscle group from virtually every angle. Whether you are targeting the chest, back, shoulders, biceps, or legs, by and large, the exercises can be done from a standing position, which is truest to real life, or from a bench or Physio Ball. We invite you to introduce cable exercises into your core workout. They are a shining example of some of the most effective and functional exercises you can use for core training. Because you are unguided through the range of motion, as is the case with other types of free weights,

UNILATERAL EQUALS ONE-SIDED

Working *unilaterally* means working one side of the body at a time. This is important because we all have a stronger side and a weaker side. Unilateral work will help create a balance between the two.

cable work affords you the added bonus of the need to summon the stabilizers into action. Working with cables with one arm or leg at a time (unilaterally) also provides the core with an extra challenge. If you are unsure of where to start, hire a trainer to help.

THE BODY PARTS Head to toe

LOWER BODY

☼ LEG PRESS MACHINE

THE FUNCTION This is an effective machine for increasing leg strength. It targets all the muscles of the legs and fully supports your back as you execute the movement. It is versatile in the sense that you are able to work unilaterally.

THE BODY PARTS Gluteals (butt), quadriceps (front upper leg), hamstrings (rear upper leg), calves (back lower leg)

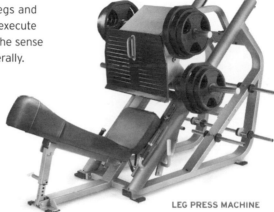

LEG PRESS MACHINE

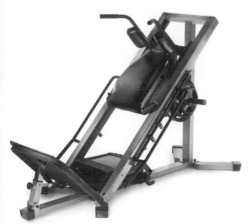

HACK SQUAT MACHINE

HACK SQUAT MACHINE

THE FUNCTION This machine works your entire lower body, putting extra emphasis on the quadriceps. An added benefit of working on this machine is that you are able to work one leg at a time (unilaterally). We all have a stronger side and a weaker side. Unilateral work will help create a balance between both sides.

THE BODY PARTS Gluteals (butt), quadriceps (front upper leg), hamstrings (rear upper leg)

133

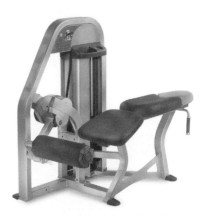

LYING HAMSTRING CURL MACHINE

HAMSTRING CURL MACHINE

THE FUNCTION Both the lying and seated versions of this machine work your hamstrings. They are equally effective. Choosing between them is strictly a matter of preference. An added benefit of working on either of these machines is that you are also able to work unilaterally.

THE BODY PARTS Hamstrings (rear upper leg)

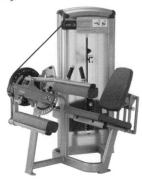

SEATED HAMSTRING CURL MACHINE

THE LOWDOWN

ADD SOME RAISES

If you're interested in using your time more efficiently, while adding some pizzazz to your work on this machine, pump out a series of calf raises in between sets.

LEG EXTENSION MACHINE

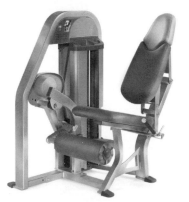

LEG EXTENSION MACHINE

THE FUNCTION This is a specialized machine strictly for working the front part of the thighs (the quadriceps). An added benefit of working on this machine is that you are able to work unilaterally.

THE BODY PARTS Quadriceps (front upper leg)

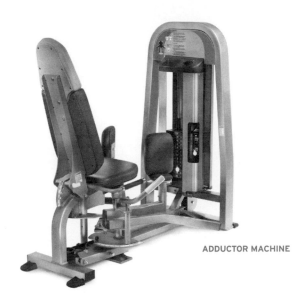

ADDUCTOR MACHINE

ADDUCTOR AND ABDUCTOR MACHINES

THE FUNCTION The adductor machine isolates the inner thighs. The abductor machine isolates the muscles that surround the hip. You will sometimes encounter one machine that is adjustable and combines the functions of these machines into one.

THE BODY PARTS Adductor machine—Adductor muscles of the inner thighs; Abductor machine—Gluteus minimus and gluteus medius (upper butt)

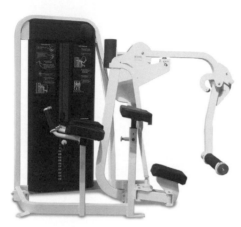

BUTT BLASTER MACHINE

BUTT BLASTER MACHINE

THE FUNCTION This machine isolates your gluteals and works the hip extenders and the back of the upper leg.

THE BODY PARTS Gluteals (butt), hamstrings (rear upper leg)

STANDING HIP MACHINE

THE FUNCTION Depending on the way you adjust the stabilizing bar and position your body, this machine is able to work all the muscles affecting your hip joint. These muscles make moving your leg in all directions possible.

THE BODY PARTS Adductors (inner thighs), abductors (upper butt), gluteals (butt), hamstrings (rear upper leg), hip flexors (front upper leg crossing the hip)

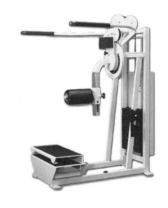

STANDING HIP MACHINE

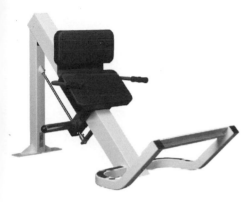

SEATED CALF MACHINE

SEATED CALF MACHINE

THE FUNCTION This works the calf muscles, especially targeting the deep part of the calf. An added benefit of working on this machine is that you are able to work unilaterally.

THE BODY PARTS Gastrocnemius (the more prominently visible calf muscle), soleus (the deep part of the calf muscles)

STANDING CALF MACHINE

THE FUNCTION This machine focuses on the more prominently visible calf muscle, and also works the deep part of the calf. An added benefit of working on this machine is that you are able to work unilaterally.

THE BODY PARTS Gastrocnemius (the more prominently seen calf muscle), soleus (the deep part of the calf muscles)

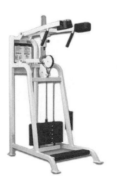

STANDING CALF MACHINE

COMBO UPPER BODY

ASSISTED PULL-UP/DIP MACHINE

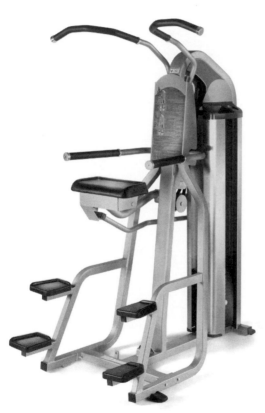

THE FUNCTION This machine can be used to do either an assisted pull-up or a triceps dip. The assisted pull-up will work the largest back muscles, the rear shoulders, and the front upper arm muscles. An added benefit of working your back with this machine is that you are able to work unilaterally. Work on this machine provides an exceptional challenge for your trunk and shoulder stabilizers.

The assisted dip will work your rear upper arm muscles, chest, and front shoulders.

The assisted pull-up/dip machine is great at helping you work toward doing a pull-up or a triceps dip with all of your body weight. It "assists" you by providing counterweight. In other words, you specify the amount of weight you'd like the machine to subtract from your body weight.

THE BODY PARTS Assisted pull-up— Latissimus dorsi (back), posterior deltoids (rear shoulders), scapular depressors; Assisted dip—Triceps (back upper arm), chest, anterior deltoids (front shoulders)

ASSISTED PULL-UP/DIP MACHINE

138

SEATED CHEST FLYE/BACK FLYE MACHINE

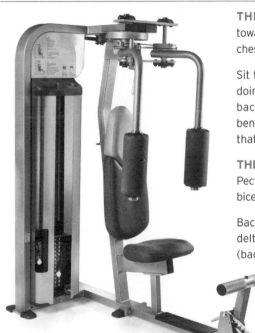

THE FUNCTION Sit with your back toward the machine and use it for doing chest flyes. This works the chest muscles.

Sit facing the machine and use it for doing back flyes, targeting your upper back and rear shoulders. An added benefit of working on this machine is that you are able to work unilaterally.

THE BODY PARTS Chest flye— Pectoralis muscles (chest muscles) and biceps (front upper arm) as stabilizers

Back flye—Upper back and posterior deltoids (rear shoulders) and triceps (back upper arm) as stabilizers

SEATED CHEST FLYE/BACK FLYE MACHINE

BACK

SEATED ROW CABLE MACHINE

THE FUNCTION This machine will work the largest back muscles that create the sculpted V-shape at your sides, as well as your rear shoulders and front upper-arm muscles. Because this machine does not provide any torso support, you'll need to recruit your core muscles to stabilize yourself while using it. An added benefit of working on this machine is that you are able to work unilaterally.

THE BODY PARTS Latissimus dorsi (back), posterior deltoids (rear shoulders), scapular retractors, spinal extensors, biceps muscles (front upper arm)

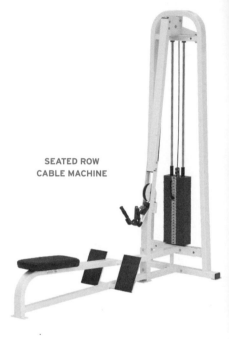

SEATED ROW CABLE MACHINE

SEATED ROW MACHINE

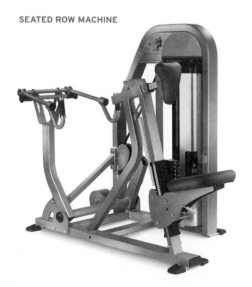

☼ SEATED ROW MACHINE

THE FUNCTION This machine will work the largest back muscles that create the sculpted V-shape at your sides, as well as your rear shoulders and front upper-arm muscles. An added benefit of working on this machine is that you are able to work unilaterally.

THE BODY PARTS Latissimus dorsi (back), posterior deltoids (rear shoulders), scapular retractors, biceps muscles (front upper arm)

INCLINE PRONE ROW MACHINE

THE FUNCTION This machine will work the largest back muscles that create the sculpted V-shape at your sides, as well as your rear shoulders and front upper-arm muscles.

THE BODY PARTS Latissimus dorsi (back), posterior deltoids (rear shoulders), scapular retractors, spinal extensors, biceps muscles (front upper arm)

INCLINE PRONE ROW MACHINE

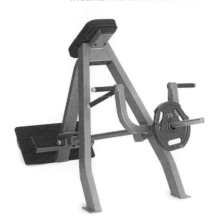

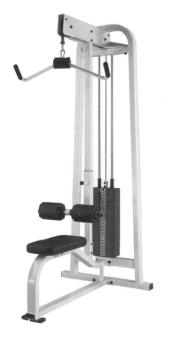

SEATED CABLE LAT PULL-DOWN MACHINE

THE FUNCTION This machine will strengthen the largest back muscles that create the sculpted V-shape at your sides, as well as your rear shoulders and front upper-arm muscles. An added benefit of working on this machine is that you are able to work unilaterally.

THE BODY PARTS Latissimus dorsi (back), posterior deltoids (rear shoulders), scapular depressors, biceps muscles (front upper arm)

SEATED CABLE LAT PULL-DOWN MACHINE

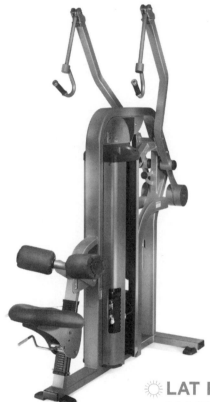

LAT PULL-DOWN MACHINE

☀ LAT PULL-DOWN MACHINE

THE FUNCTION This machine will strengthen the largest back muscles that create the sculpted V-shape at your sides, as well as your rear shoulders and front upper-arm muscles. An added benefit of working on this machine is that you are able to work unilaterally.

THE BODY PARTS Latissimus dorsi (back), posterior deltoids (rear shoulders), scapular depressors, biceps muscles (front upper arm)

CHEST

☼ CHEST PRESS MACHINE

THE FUNCTION The chest press machine targets the chest muscles as well as the front shoulders and rear upper-arm muscles. An added benefit of working on this machine is that you are able to work unilaterally.

THE BODY PARTS Pectoralis muscles (chest), anterior deltoids (front shoulders), triceps muscles (rear upper arm)

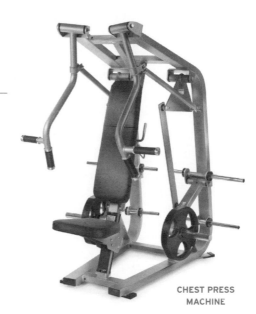

CHEST PRESS
MACHINE

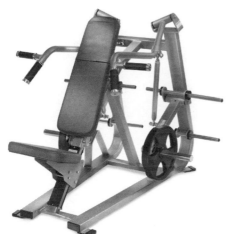

INCLINE CHEST PRESS MACHINE

INCLINE CHEST PRESS MACHINE

THE FUNCTION This machine will target the chest muscles. Because you are pushing up on an angle, you will be putting emphasis on the upper region of the chest. It will also work the front shoulders and rear upper-arm muscles. An added benefit of working on this machine is that you are able to work unilaterally.

THE BODY PARTS Pectoralis muscles (chest), anterior deltoids (front shoulders), triceps muscles (rear upper arm)

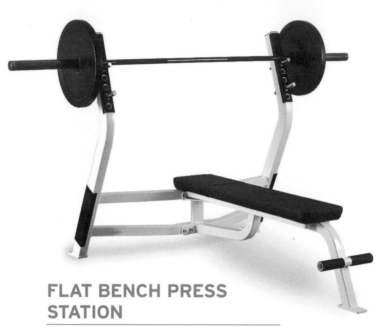

FLAT BENCH PRESS STATION

THE FUNCTION The bench press targets the chest muscles as well as the front shoulders and rear upper-arm muscles. Because you are using a free weight, you are fully in charge of guiding the bar through the exercise and get the added benefit of working the stabilizers of the shoulders. Performing a chest press on a flat bench is more advanced and arguably also more rewarding than doing it on the chest press machine for this reason. Once you master the machine, try this exercise. The two are interchangeable.

THE BODY PARTS Pectoralis muscles (chest), anterior deltoids (front shoulders), triceps muscles (rear upper arm)

FLAT BENCH PRESS STATION

INCLINE BENCH PRESS STATION

THE FUNCTION The chest muscles will be the focus of this exercise. Pushing up on an angle will put more emphasis on the upper region of the chest. This exercise will also work the front shoulders and rear upper arm muscles. Because you are using a free weight, you are fully in charge of guiding the bar through the exercise and get the added benefit of working the stabilizers of the shoulders. Performing an incline chest press on an incline bench is more advanced, and arguably also more rewarding, than doing it on the incline chest press machine for this reason. Once you master the machine, try this exercise. The two are interchangeable.

THE BODY PARTS Pectoralis muscles (chest), anterior deltoids (front shoulders), triceps muscles (rear upper arm)

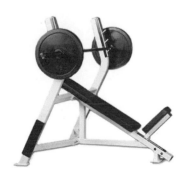

INCLINE BENCH PRESS STATION

SHOULDERS

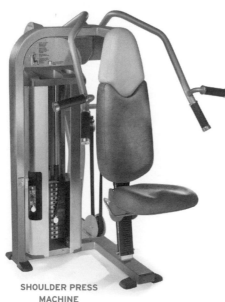

SHOULDER PRESS MACHINE

☼ SHOULDER PRESS MACHINE

THE FUNCTION This machine will work the front shoulders, the more prominent muscle of the upper back, and the rear upper-arm muscles. An added benefit of working on this machine is that you are able to work unilaterally.

THE BODY PARTS Anterior deltoids (front shoulder), trapezius muscle (upper back), triceps muscles (rear upper arm)

☼ LATERAL RAISE MACHINE

THE FUNCTION The sides of your shoulders are the target when working on this machine. An added benefit of working on this machine is that you are able to work unilaterally.

THE BODY PARTS Medial deltoids (side of the shoulders)

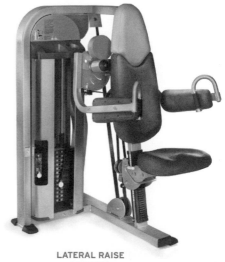

LATERAL RAISE MACHINE

BICEPS

BICEPS MACHINE

THE FUNCTION The muscles in the front part of your upper arm (commonly referred to as the "guns") are targeted with this machine.

THE BODY PARTS Biceps muscles (front upper arm)

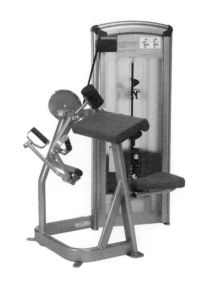

BICEPS MACHINE

TRICEPS

TRICEPS MACHINE

THE FUNCTION The muscles in the rear part of your upper arm are targeted with this machine.

THE BODY PARTS Triceps muscles (rear upper arm)

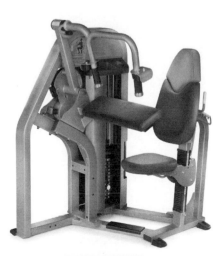

TRICEPS MACHINE

CORE

ROMAN CHAIR

THE FUNCTION The most popular exercise on this machine strengthens the lower back, as well as the glutes and backs of the upper legs. You can also shift positions so that you are side-lying on the machine and, in addition to the lower back, work the core muscles in the front and sides of the body

THE BODY PARTS Erector spinae (lower back), rectus abdominus (six-pack), obliques (side abdominals), gluteals (butt), hamstrings (rear upper leg)

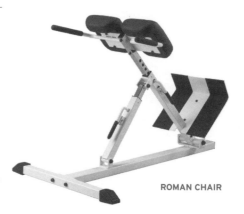

ROMAN CHAIR

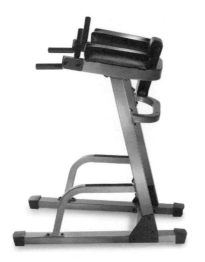

CAPTAIN'S CHAIR

CAPTAIN'S CHAIR

THE FUNCTION This stand, which resembles a seatless high chair, is used to work the lower region of the abdominal muscles as well as the front of the hips and upper leg. Your lower chest, side, back, and rear shoulder muscles work as stabilizers. It's also used as a tool to work the rear upper-arm muscles.

THE BODY PARTS Iliopsoas (hip flexor), rectus femoris (front upper leg), rectus abdominus (six-pack), obliques (side abdominals), pectoralis muscles (chest), latissimus dorsi (back), posterior deltoids (rear shoulders), triceps muscles (rear upper arm)

ROTARY TORSO MACHINE

THE FUNCTION This machine works the side abdominal muscles.

THE BODY PARTS Obliques (side abdominals)

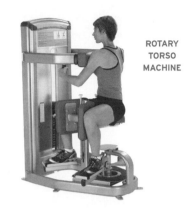

ROTARY TORSO MACHINE

AB SLING (REVERSE CRUNCH HANGING STRAPS)

THE FUNCTION These straps are used to work the lower region of the abdominal muscles as well as the front of the hips and upper leg. Your lower chest, side, back, and rear shoulder muscles work as stabilizers. Extra control is required in order to avoid using the help of momentum when working with this piece of equipment.

THE BODY PARTS Iliopsoas (hip flexor), rectus femoris (front upper leg), rectus abdominus (six-pack), obliques (side abdominals), pectoralis muscles (chest), latissimus dorsi (back), posterior deltoids (back shoulders)

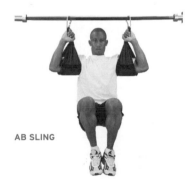

AB SLING

TORSO CURL MACHINE

THE FUNCTION Your abdominal muscles are strengthened through the use of this machine.

THE BODY PARTS Rectus abdominus (six-pack), obliques (side abdominals)

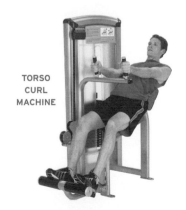

TORSO CURL MACHINE

149

CARDIOVASCULAR EQUIPMENT

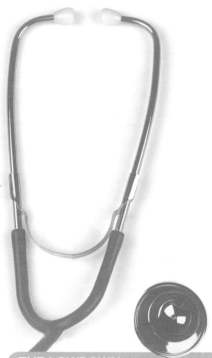

The primary purpose for doing cardiovascular work is to train the most important muscle in your body—your heart. Many pieces of cardiovascular equipment are designed to mimic outdoor activities (running, climbing, cycling, etc.), often *sans* the joint-jarring high-impact aspect of the exercise (elliptical machines, the Arc Trainer). Others are simply designed to get you moving (usually, your legs) in order to get your heart rate up. By sharing a few details about yourself with the machine (gender, age, and weight), it is able to monitor your workout and provide feedback on interesting and noteworthy information such as your heart rate, speed, distance, power (watts), time, and calories burned. The machines act somewhat like automated personal trainers, offering a wide range of training profiles to keep your workouts varied (and boredom-free as a bonus). Some of the profiles you can expect to encounter are hills, intervals, competitions, and random (a mix of most). You will usually have the option of creating your own personalized format by selecting the "manual" setting on the machine as well.

THE LOWDOWN

CONTROVERSIAL CALORIE COUNTING

The calorie-counting feature on cardiovascular machines is commonly followed with dogmatic vigilance, and is sometimes even believed to be the true measure of the success of a workout. Because of this, we feel it is necessary to point out the rudimentary fact that often it is not being totally sincere with you. This information should always be taken lightly. Although it is useful and should not be trivialized, consider that the calorie counter doesn't know you personally. It doesn't take into account vital information such as your fat-to-muscle ratio or how fit you currently are. The machine will not be able to tell you precisely how many calories *your* body burns at the particular level of activity you have chosen. If you are interested in a more accurate calorie-burning count, see a personal trainer.

Gyms have so many different pieces of cardiovascular equipment; you may be wondering how to choose which is best for you. Are some better than others? Which is most effective? There is no perfect answer to these questions; they depend on your specific fitness goals, physical conditions, and personal preferences. For example, from the calorie-burning point of view, running is a good way to go. If you don't enjoy running, however, you'd probably work more passionately and burn more calories working on something you really had an affinity for. If you have vulnerable joints, it is also probably not the activity we would advocate. Conversely, if you are training for a marathon, aside from a road outdoors, the treadmill should be your best friend.

We often see people working on the same type of cardiovascular machine on a daily basis. Often this is because they have truly fallen in love with this particular machine. Mingling with other pieces of equipment is very healthy. There is much to be said for cross-training. It will allow you to develop strength in different skills and limit the possibilities of overuse injuries. Be adventurous, and every now and then, try a different machine.

THE LOWDOWN

MINDLESS

We all love a good book or racy television show, but there is a time and place for everything, and the gym is not the place to spend time catching up on your reading or your favorite sitcom. We often notice folks engrossed in a novel or watching their favorite soap opera while using cardio equipment. Their legs are often moving so slowly, you almost want to tap them on the shoulder to make sure they are still conscious and haven't been hypnotized by their TV show or book. Their minds are completely disconnected from the activity their bodies are supposed to be engaged in. We guarantee that you will get much more out of your workout in a shorter amount of time if you are present and focused (this goes for anything you do in life, by the way). Your workout will be much more fun and effective. Plus, it may prevent you from sliding right off the treadmill and embarrassing yourself. (We've seen it happen.)

HEART START

For the newcomer to cardiovascular training, here are some simple guidelines to get you going. If you are really serious about this and can afford it, we counsel you to hire a personal trainer who can help design a program that is specific to your goals and needs.

To begin with, schedule two to three days a week for your cardio workouts. Each workout should last 20 to 30 minutes at an easy-to-moderate intensity. At a moderate intensity, you will definitely feel a change in your breath rate. It is an intensity that you are able to sustain for longer periods of time with noticeable but tolerable discomfort. Realize this will only get you started. In time your body will adapt to this workout and be ready for a greater challenge.

This greater challenge can be achieved by doing one of three things: increasing the amount of time spent on the machine, increasing the intensity, or increasing the number of days you do the workout. Be sure to build on only one of these elements at a time, and only in small increments. For example, increase the time you spend working on a machine by five minutes, without changing the intensity or the number of workouts in a week.

Another example would be to do the same workout you had been doing one additional day per week.

Make minor adjustments to your workout about every couple of weeks or so. Small, consistent steps are the safest and most effective ways to make progress. If after six weeks you realize you have not made any changes, avoid the temptation of making a drastic change. Limit your adjustment to somewhere between 5 and 10 percent. For example, if you were running 2 miles regularly, increase your distance to 2.2 miles. Once you reach your ultimate aspired cardiovascular destination (this may sound obvious), level off. Your focus will shift from gaining to maintaining. If you take more than two weeks off from your training, note that you will have to scale back to an easy-to-moderate level and build up to where you once were. Don't worry; now that you have built a base, you will bounce back quickly. Training is an ongoing journey.

THE LOWDOWN

CARDIO CONFINEMENTS

During the busiest hours, some gyms will set time limits for some of the cardiovascular equipment. In these cases you will have to sign up and possibly wait in line for an available machine.

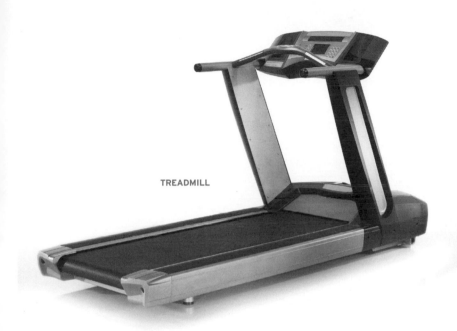

TREADMILL

TREADMILL

THE FUNCTION This all-time favorite cardiovascular machine will simulate a walking, jogging, or running experience along a multitude of terrains ranging from a long, flat road to a steep mountain path, or various combinations of both. On most treadmills you'll have the ability to use time, distance, or calories as a means of measuring the extent of your session. (Sprinkle a grain or two of salt on the calorie-burning readouts. They are usually quantitatively tasteless. See "The

Lowdown" on page 150.) The running bed (the rubberized platform under your feet) is usually fitted with a suspension system, lessening the high-impact effects outdoor running can have on the joints.

> A treadmill is suitable for anyone, depending on the activity of choice. Those with healthy joints can run their hearts wild, but although the treadmill will remove some of the jarring effects outdoor running can have on the joints, it is not the best prescription for those with weak or previously injured backs, knees, ankles, or hips. Such individuals are better off walking or jogging lightly on the treadmill, or working out on less joint-jolting, low-impact machines such as the stationary bike or one of the stair climbers.

STAIRMASTER

THE FUNCTION The concept behind this machine is simple. Working on a StairMaster is meant to mimic climbing stairs, as its name implies. While you'll never be lifting your feet completely off the pedals to climb up as you would with climbing actual stairs, the pedals are designed as gait simulators, ergonomically mimicking the natural movement of your body as it climbs. You'll be given the option of choosing between several preset profiles that modify the resistance and incline of each step or manually creating your own.

> This machine provides a low-impact cardio workout that can be adapted to people of all levels of conditioning.

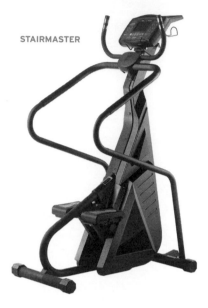

STAIRMASTER

STAIR MILL
MACHINE

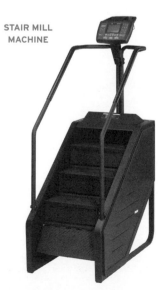

STAIR MILL MACHINE

THE FUNCTION As with the StairMaster, the Stair Mill is another stand-in for climbing stairs. It more closely resembles stairs as we know them in life because it simulates a revolving staircase. Because you'll be lifting each foot off one step and onto another moving step, it requires heightened focus.

> This machine provides a low-impact cardio workout that can be adapted to people of all levels of conditioning. Start out at a slow pace until you become better acquainted with the motion. Be willing to pay close attention to your every step on this machine every time you are using it, regardless of your level of Stair Mill savvy.

STATIONARY BICYCLE

THE FUNCTION A stationary bike is a stand-in for riding a real outdoor bicycle. You will discover that most gyms will have two particular types of stationary bikes. One is the standard upright model, and the other is the recumbent bike, where you are seated with your legs pedaling out in front of you. Riding a stationary bike is a great way to remove all the elements you would be forced to face when riding outdoors and ensure a precise training session. For example, indoors there is no chance of plans being thwarted by the weather's capricious tendencies. With a stationary bike you become the virtual architect of the exact road you desire for your training and eliminate the extra time and effort you would otherwise need to dedicate to finding that road outdoors.

STATIONARY
BICYCLE

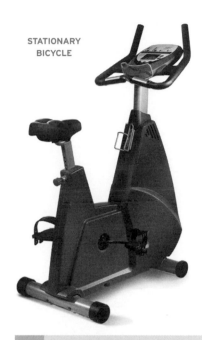

THE LOWDOWN

STAIR SKILLS

If the StairMaster is bearing most of your weight over its handrails and your legs are stepping lightly on the pedals, you can extrapolate without much doubt that you are not going to gain much from doing this exercise. Unless you're skilled in the practice of levitation, and when confronted by a set of stairs can hover up to the top, this is not the intended exercise. Remember, this should feel like you are actually climbing stairs. You should feel most of the weight of your body on the pedals.

> Both models are capable of stepping up to the plate and responding dutifully when presented with an honest effort. Because of the likeness in aerodynamic positioning of some upright models, they're the closest relative of an outdoor bicycle and therefore reflect a more realistic experience. Holding that position for an extended period of time requires keeping an engaged core, and may otherwise aggravate your lower back. The recumbent bike is easier on the lower back. Some people also find the wider, more chairlike seat of a recumbent bicycle easier to tolerate and less offensive to the nether areas of the body than the saddle of the upright model. The recumbent bike, however, has been accused of coercing increased soreness to the hips and legs.

155

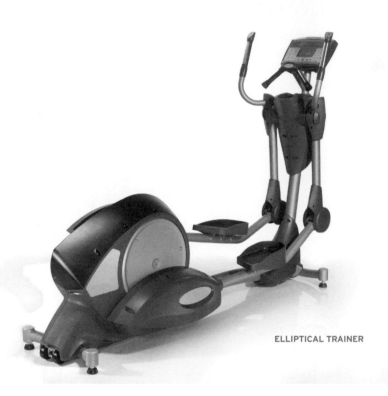

ELLIPTICAL TRAINER

ELLIPTICAL TRAINER

THE FUNCTION The Elliptical Trainer is a hybrid of a treadmill and a StairMaster. This machine is another example of a gait simulator in that the elliptical range of motion of the pedals simulates the natural range of motion of our legs when we walk, jog, or run. It is unique in its ability to fuse a nonimpact form of cardiovascular exercise with a weight-bearing activity.

Your bones respond to weight by becoming stronger and weight-bearing exercises are the secret to preemptively striking the possibility of developing osteoporosis in years to come. (A much more effective preemptive strike against developing osteoporosis, and also nonimpact, is

 The Elliptical Trainer is user friendly and a good option for all populations.

CROSS-COUNTRY SKI MACHINE

THE FUNCTION The level of athleticism required to propel your body along snow-veiled paths on skis is immensely vigorous for the cardiovascular system, muscles of the upper and lower body, and joints. This machine's intent is to bring that outdoor, often frigid experience to the temperate indoors. Cross-country ski machines offer a great low-impact full-body workout and are a great way to practice the sport as a beginner without running the risk of exhausting yourself and getting stuck in a cold and obscure place. Once you have completed your session or don't feel like you are able to glide on any longer, just stop and you are free to go.

> Some cross-country ski machines are better than others, offering the option to modify the incline to simulate uphill climbs and other varied terrain, as well as separate resistance controls for its lower- and upper-body components.

THE LOWDOWN

THE ORIGINAL SKIER

The first cross-country ski machine was introduced by the company Icon Fitness in the 1980s and is called the NordicTrack.

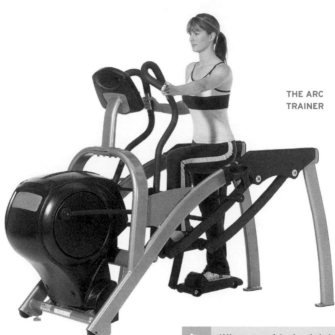

THE ARC
TRAINER

THE ARC TRAINER

THE FUNCTION Similar to the Elliptical Trainer, the Arc Trainer is another example of a gait simulator by virtue of the fact that it deliberately guides you through your natural range of motion when walking, jogging, or running without requiring your feet to ever leave the surface of the foot platforms. In this case, the range of motion forms the shape of an arc rather than an ellipse. The benefits associated with the Arc Trainer are the same as those of the Elliptical Trainer.

> When considering joint preservation, protecting them from the damaging jolts caused by high-impact activities is the first thing to come to mind. There is, however, another, often overlooked yet unequivocally critical component to consider. This is the possible tweak or torque of your joints by moving in unnatural ranges of motion. The Arc Trainer is a newer piece of equipment than the Elliptical Trainer, and there are some studies that claim that the arcing range of motion is more synchronous to that of natural movement than the ellipse, and is therefore less stress-inducing to the joints. Seeing as we all have different types of bodies, try both and see what fits you best.

ROWING MACHINE

THE FUNCTION The function of this machine is quite straightforward. It attempts to reflect rowing as an outdoor water sport, and for that matter, is quite successful, offering parallel benefits. At comparable levels of intensity, the rowing machine is recognized as one of the greatest calorie-burning pieces of equipment at the gym. It is a machine that engages almost all of the major muscle groups and rolls cardiovascular training and strength conditioning into one.

> Rowing is an activity that can be enjoyed at any age or fitness level. It is a nonimpact activity and great for rehabilitative purposes as well.

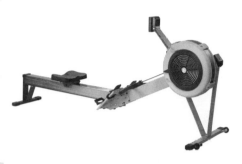

ROWING MACHINE

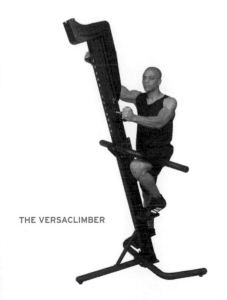

THE VERSACLIMBER

THE VERSACLIMBER

THE FUNCTION The VersaClimber will give you the experience of an unrelenting alfresco rock climb along with all of the related full-body cardio and strength conditioning benefits. While your lower body engages in a stepping motion, your upper body pushes and pulls, mobilizing your arms vertically above your head. This is a feature unique to the VersaClimber, as most other cardiovascular machines simulate horizontal movement. A workout on the VersaClimber will challenge all the major muscle groups in a nonimpact motion.

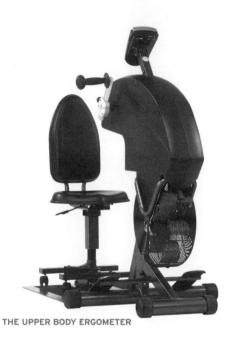

THE UPPER BODY ERGOMETER

THE UPPER-BODY ERGOMETER

THE FUNCTION Sometimes referred to as a tabletop or upper-body bike, a workout on this machine can be interpreted as cycling with your arms. It is one of the only upper body–isolating cardio machines in existence. Like a stationary bike, it allows you to select the amount of resistance your upper body will need to contend with.

> This machine is a phenomenal innovation and worthy of applause because of the allure it has to those with any type of lower-body injury or those who are in the midst of rehabilitation. Exercising on this machine will minimally impact your joints while strengthening your upper body. It is also a great way to warm up before an upper-body strength training session.

THE LOWDOWN

CARDIO CALCULATIONS

Have a very specific plan when you use a piece of cardio equipment. Creating a program with different goals for each cardio workout will help you get the most out of your workout and make time seem like it's flying.

CARDIO GAMES

There are days when you wake up in the morning with rays of sun radiating brightly through your window. The birds are chirping sweet songs in the background, and you know you're "on" for the day. You feel like no matter what you decide to do, it will work out famously. Then there are other days. Everything feels wrong and you are swimming upstream all day and no matter what the task, it is a struggle. When you're just not into it, any amount of time doing a cardiovascular workout can be brutal and may seem to last forever. Skipping a planned workout, on the other hand, may hollow out your heart, and leave you with nothing but feelings of self-defeat. Here are a couple of our own personal "games" that help get us through those tough days. They work flawlessly on the "good" days as added elements of intrigue as well.

PUSH THE PACE GAME

This game will work on any piece of cardiovascular equipment. Warm up for 5 to 10 minutes. By the end of your warm-up, you should begin to feel slightly sweat-moistened, and comfortably challenged. Speed up your pace. You should go fast enough to feel a noticeable difference in your speed while maintaining proper form. Hold this quick pace for three to five minutes. This should be difficult to maintain and you should be breathing pretty heavily. Slow back down to your moderate pace for an equal amount of time in order to recover. Allow yourself to fully catch your breath before repeating the speed interval. Repeat three to six times.

THE UPHILL CHALLENGE

This game also works on any piece of equipment. Warm up for 5 to 10 minutes. By the end of your warm-up, you should begin to feel slightly sweat-moistened, and comfortably challenged. Keep the same pace or cadence and increase your incline (or resistance) to step up your effort from moderate or kind of hard to very hard. Keep the resistance at that level for three to five minutes. Holding this should feel difficult and you should be breathing pretty heavily. Lower the resistance back down to your moderate level for an equal amount of time to recover. Allow yourself to fully catch your breath before climbing your next hill. Repeat three to six times.

161

Both of these games will help fill out a good chunk of time. They can be full cardio workouts on their own or can be sandwiched by longer stretches of endurance work at a less intense pace. Don't forget to dedicate another 5 to 10 minutes or so to a cool down.

These cardio games will oblige you to keep your mind on your workouts and make them fly by in the blink of an eye.

You will have given yourself a kick-butt workout, earning tomorrow as a lighter or recovery day. You will also be guiltlessly free to move on to other interesting things (like another type of workout, or a soothing massage). This by itself is certainly enough to get your blood circulating, and heck, may even be enough to circulate the dark cloud right out of your day.

MENTAL MOTIVATORS

Use the exponential power of the mind to your advantage. If you're able to guide your thoughts in a positive and motivating direction throughout your workout, your body will respond accordingly. See below for a few ways to do this.

Keep a clear picture of your fitness goals in your mind's eye. Remind yourself that the activity you are doing is what will help you get there. Actually envision yourself as if you have already reached your goals. How does it feel to be perfectly healthy and stronger than ever? What do you look like?

Bring your attention to the rhythm of your breathing. Inhale deeply and feel your breath traveling through your body and filling it with energy. Exhale and feel any tension you are experiencing being carried out of your body with your breath.

Allow yourself to feel what is going on in your body. Scan your body for tension, especially around the shoulders and neck. Let go of that tension. During the toughest efforts, when you feel assaulted by intense feelings of discomfort, don't fight it by clenching your muscles. Notice these feeling, don't judge them, and allow them to flow freely through your body. Bringing your attention back to breathing may help.

CORE STRENGTH, BALANCE, AND STABILITY EQUIPMENT

Besides the strength training equipment designed to target the abdominal domain, most gyms will be furnished with a plethora of free-standing, non-machine-like tools to help tone up your core muscles and improve your balance and stability. Judging by the amount of new equipment popping up in the market these days, we suspect that there are round-the-clock think tanks conceptualizing new ab-fortifying contraptions in secret locations around the world. We have done our best to include as many as possible, but by the time this book hits mass markets, we bet there will be some that will have been sadly omitted. We invite you to cast your reservations aside and try as many of these tools as possible. The payoff for integrating a melange of exercises using a variety of different tools is nothing less than well-rounded core strength and fine-tuned balance and stability.

AB WHEEL

THE FUNCTION Every muscle of the core falls prey to the Ab Wheel, and will be fully charged and challenged from its use. This is a tool for very advanced exercises also requiring extra engagement of the muscles of the lower back. Here is a simple example of a very advanced exercise using the wheel. Hold on to the grips fitted on either side of the wheel. Push the wheel out in front of you, bracing all the muscles of your core to control the movement and to keep your hips from sagging, and roll back to starting position. The exercise can be done from the knees or toes. From the toes, this exercise becomes even more sophisticated and extra challenging.

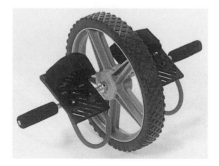

AB WHEEL

AB DOLLY

THE FUNCTION The Ab Dolly is an upgraded derivative of the Ab Wheel. The rolling out concept is the same, but the Dolly is a multihandled platform on wheels, and is more versatile. You're able to roll out from your arms or place the Dolly under your knees and roll your lower body in and out. When you become a Dolly virtuoso, try using two Dollies, one under each arm or each knee. This will allow you to work on balancing both sides of your body and further challenge your coordination.

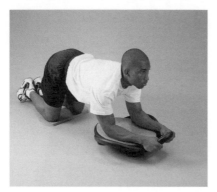

AB DOLLY

BALANCE PILLOW

THE FUNCTION Balance pillows are air-filled discs used for creating a volatile surface on which to practice balance; ankle, knee, hip, and shoulder stability; and proprioception training. There are many different varieties of balance pillows available. The smaller pillows are optimal for placing under each foot, knee, or hand. Just about any exercise normally done on the floor can be performed on a balance pillow(s).

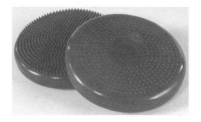

BALANCE PILLOW

INTERNAL COMPASS

Proprioception is the body's ability to sense its own spatial position, location, orientation, and movement.

WOBBLE BOARDS

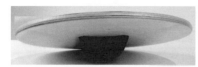

WOBBLE BOARDS

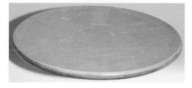

THE FUNCTION Though varying in shapes and sizes, all wobble boards basically serve the same purpose. Through their wobbling, they make any exercise done while standing on them more challenging by rivaling your balancing skills. Working on them will help build ankle, knee, and hip stability and work overall balance and coordination. The boards can also be used for push-ups and planks, and as a "bench" for chest presses and flyes, for example. They are quite versatile. Use your imagination. To make the most out of your gym time, keep a wobble board close by and use it in between sets.

REEBOK CORE BOARD

THE FUNCTION Essentially, this is a wobble board with an added feature. It is fitted with a lever that allows you to control its level of stability. This is great for those who are unaccustomed to working on wobble boards or any other type of stability-challenging tool.

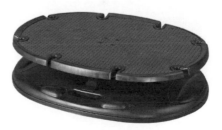

CORE BOARD

VEW-DO BOARD

THE FUNCTION This board, bearing a close resemblance to the well-known skate board, will put to the test your balance, coordination, stabilizing, and proprioceptive skills. The board rests on a roller that will move from side to side, and in the more advanced versions, also rock forward and backward. Your challenge is to maintain your balance while the board moves underneath you. Once you are able to hold your balance on the Vew-Do Board, try squats, and shoulder presses

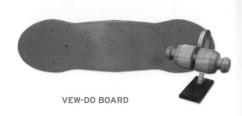

VEW-DO BOARD

(and any other standing exercises) while standing on one. You can also try to balance on the board with your arms and do straight arm planks and push-ups.

PHYSIO BALL

THE FUNCTION This oversized air-filled ball, sometimes referred to as the Swiss Ball or Resist-a-Ball, allows traditional ab exercises to be done with a fuller range of motion than when performed on the floor. Its roundness creates instability and beckons a formidable balance act from your body. In adapting to this unsteady playing field, the body learns to react quickly and accurately. The Physio Ball can act as a substitute for a bench and add balance and stability challenges to almost any free weight exercise and is also immensely versatile when used alone.

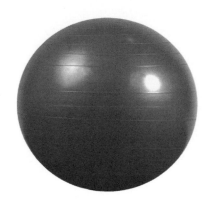

PHYSIO BALL

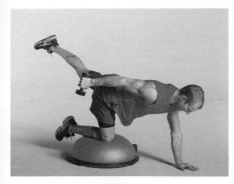

BOSU

BOSU

THE FUNCTION The BOSU, which stands for "both sides up," is a combination of the Physio Ball and wobble boards. Because it is half a ball, fitted on a solid platform, and not freely rolling around, it is easier to stand on than the Physio Ball (although standing on a Physio Ball is possible with practice as well). Perform the exercises you would with either a Physio Ball or wobble boards on a BOSU for improved balance, stability, and coordination. The possibilities are virtually endless.

MEDICINE BALL

THE FUNCTION Medicine balls are available in a variety of different weights and sizes ranging from 1 through 30 pounds. Some are plain round balls, while others have a fancy handle (or handles) built into them to facilitate grip. The entire motley crew of medicine balls, whether simple or adorned with extra details, present a safe and fun way to add weight to your training. The ways in which to use them in a workout border on infinite (far too many to elaborate in detail in this book), and it is a good idea to talk to a trainer or invest in a book exclusively dedicated to the topic. For example, it can be as easy as simply holding one while doing a basic crunch or throwing one back and forth with a partner or trainer. You can use them to add

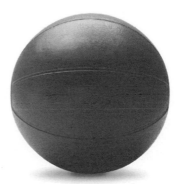

MEDICINE BALL

weight as well as a coordination challenge to twists, chops, and a number of other dynamic, full-body exercises emphasizing the core. For a balance challenge, try standing on a medicine ball or using it in conjunction with a wobble board.

BANDS/TUBING

THE FUNCTION Rubber bands and tubing, akin to cables in function, are great strength training tools. While in portability they are more versatile than cables, the level of resistance throughout the range of motion is not as consistent. The farther away you pull the bands or tubing, the greater the resistance. This type of equipment is also an excellent option for a home gym, where space may be limited. It has the capacity to offer a comprehensive, full-body workout.

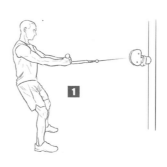

BANDS

TUBING

CABLES

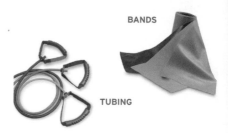

1

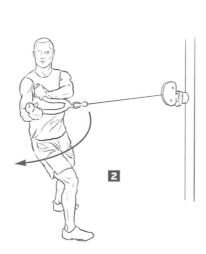

2

HORIZONTAL ROTATION

THE CABLE CORE CAPTIVATOR

Cables are highly exalted in our book. Here's an example of a challenging and dynamic way we use them to strengthen our core muscles in a useful-in-the-real-world sort of way. Below we offer you a cable teaser. We prompt you to enlist the help of a trainer to show you in greater detail how to get started with these exercises, and a bunch more.

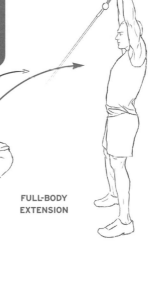

FULL-BODY EXTENSION

1

3D CRUNCH

2

3

ADJUSTABLE AB BENCH

THE FUNCTION This bench can be adjusted to several different levels of incline. This enables you to vary the level of intensity in which you execute many abdominal exercises. For example, doing a basic crunch on a platform with your rear end positioned higher than your torso is much more difficult than doing the same exercise on a flat plane. This bench can also be used as a strength training bench or platform. Be creative with it.

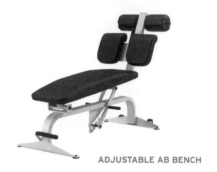

ADJUSTABLE AB BENCH

URBAN REBOUNDER

THE FUNCTION The soft surface of this mini-trampoline is not only meant for bouncing around. The instability it provides creates a balance challenge, firing up all of the body's stabilizers when anyone is standing or kneeling on it with one or both legs. It can also be used as a mat for core work, a surface for non-joint-jarring plyometric work, and a cardio workout tool.

URBAN REBOUNDER

ANCILLARY EQUIPMENT

Details are often what make the difference between the ordinary and the exceptional. That extra touch is what can crown an overall experience. It is the ancillary equipment that will accessorize your workout. Ancillary equipment such as platforms and dumbbell racks is likely to be found at most clubs, while others such as the BodyWedge21, and Kettlebells may not be. Some of the equipment listed below, such as butterfly clips and bar pads, will work in conjunction with other equipment to make your workouts more safe and comfortable.

PLYOBOXES

PLATFORMS

THE FUNCTION For a quick and easy way to manipulate the vertical plane you're working on, platforms are ideal. They are available in many different heights and, in addition to being a tool for simple step-ups, are great for performing plyometric drills. Low platforms can be a fun addition to some quickness drills as well.

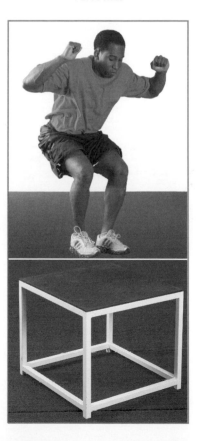

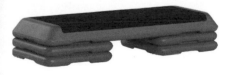

PLATFORMS

GYM SURVIVAL GUIDE

PLATFORM MOVES

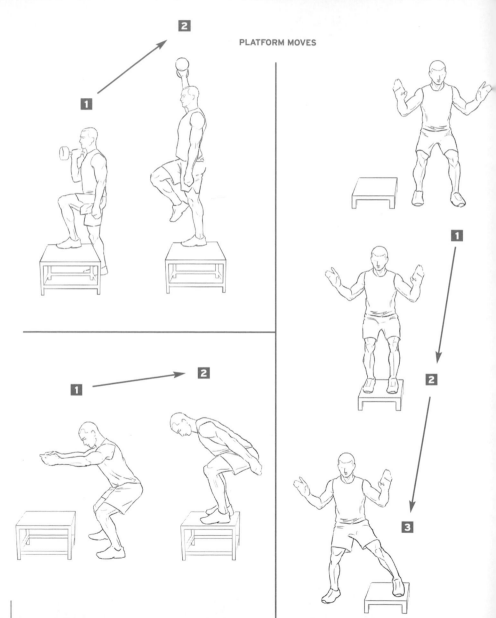

DUMBBELL RACK

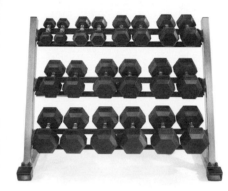

DUMBBELL RACK

THE FUNCTION These will usually be found in the form of a tower or a long, horizontal multi-level shelving unit. In the horizontal configuration, the higher levels will normally house the lighter weights and the lower, the heavier weights. The weights will also be arranged in order from lightest to heaviest from left to right and generally range from 5, 8, 12, and 15 to 100 pounds (the weights in between 15 and 100 pounds usually escalate in 5-pound increments).

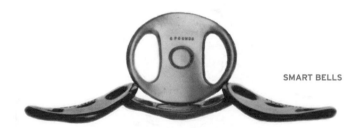

SMART BELLS

SMART BELLS

THE FUNCTION Smart Bells are weights uniquely designed to conform to the shape of your body while remaining balanced through flowing movement. They are revolutionary in that they hold a copyright as a sculpture, as well as a patent for their unique ergonomic form and signature circular Smart Bell movement patterns.

The concept behind the Smart Bell is to encourage "effortless and synergistic" weight-assisted movement. While tradi-tional exercises can also be done using the Smart Bells, the patented three-minute Smart Bells Routine is designed to capture the flowing movements much akin to those of a Sun Salutation or Tai Chi.

Smart Bells were sculpted and patented by Paul Widerman, former Captain of the Harvard Wrestling Team and U.S. Olympic Team Alternate. You can see more at www.THINKFIT.com.

BODY BARS

THE FUNCTION Body Bars are colorfully capped, rubber-covered weighted steel bars. They are extremely versatile and can be used for practically any exercise. (Check out our book *Body Bar: 133 Moves for Full-Body Fitness,*) They are available in a variety of weights ranging from 3 to 36 pounds.

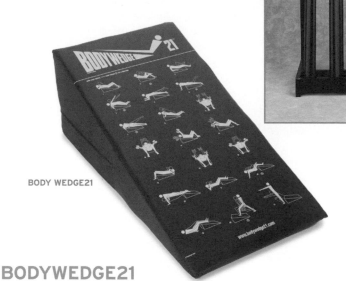

BODY WEDGE21

BODY BARS

BODYWEDGE21

THE FUNCTION The BodyWedge21 is designed to be an exercise ball, step, and incline/decline bench all rolled into one. Its soft, foam-filled surface offers a stability challenge, while its shape acts as a platform and sloping ramp. So, what is the 21 all about? The surface of this slice of foam-filled fun is illustrated with 21 exercises. These exercises were created specifically for the BodyWedge21 and destined to fire up the abdominals, gluteals, thighs, chest, and lower back. The Wedge can be used alone for performing exercises using only your body weight, or in conjunction with bands, hand weights, medicine balls, and the like.

KETTLEBELLS

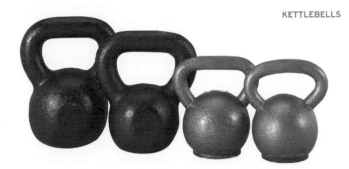

KETTLEBELL

THE FUNCTION A Kettlebell is a cast iron-handled ball used for total body strengthenin, and toning of the muscles. Kettlebells, now made with a softer rubberized exterior, can also be used to add intensity to cardio workouts. They are available in a wide range of weights, making them a great tool for people of all levels of fitness. Kettlebell training is an ancient Russian method of exercise, long recognized by the likes of Russian Olympic champions and Soviet Special Forces, to help develop agility, strength, and stamina. Talk to a trainer to learn how to use them.

JUMP ROPE

THE FUNCTION For your own personal training, or jump rope- and/or boxing-related classes, most clubs will have an assortment of jump ropes available for your use. They're wonderful tools for developing speed, agility, and endurance.

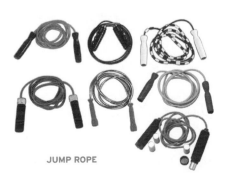

JUMP ROPE

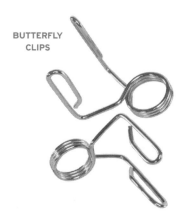

BUTTERFLY
CLIPS

BUTTERFLY CLIPS OR OLYMPIC SPRING COLLARS

THE FUNCTION These springy clips are safety clips. They attach onto the ends of the Olympic bars in order to secure the plates onto them. Should you accidentally tip the bar over to one side, you won't run the risk of dropping the plates on yourself or on some unsuspecting passerby.

BAR PADS

THE FUNCTION Bar pads are vinyl-covered foam pads that wrap around the Olympic bar or Smith Machine bar in order to cushion your neck from their weight. They are usually found somewhere in the vicinity of the squat rack or Smith machine and can easily be secured on the bars with their Velcro closures. You may also encounter what is called a Manta Ray. This basically serves the same purpose, easing neck discomfort, but does so by acting as a weight distributor. It will apportion the weight from your neck across your trapezius muscles. The Manta Ray will snap on to the bar, instead of wrapping around it.

BAR PADS

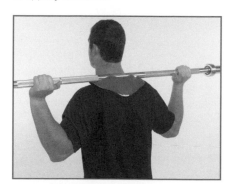

FLEXIBILITY- AND STRETCHING-SPECIFIC EQUIPMENT

There are several pieces of equipment available at most gyms to help you isolate those hard-to-stretch areas. Following are a few. It is a definite plus to learn how to use them.

FOAM ROLLER

THE FUNCTION This is the perfect self-massaging tool. It is mostly used for releasing tension or tightness in muscles and connective tissue. It is especially useful for relaxing the IT band (the IT band begins at the top of the hip and runs all the way down to your knee on the side of your leg), which when tight and uncared for can lead to afflictions in the knee and hip.

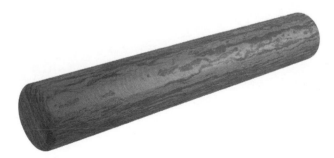

FOAM ROLLER

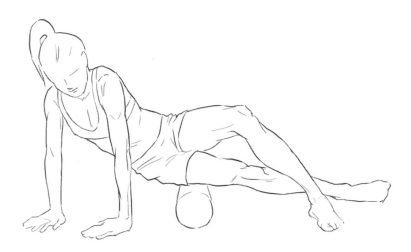

To work on the IT band, lie on your side with the foam roller just below your hip. Shift your weight with your arms and legs on the floor in order to adjust the amount of pressure on the IT band. Slowly move your body toward your head, and let the foam roller roll down the outside of your leg until it is just above the side of your knee. You can also roll out any other muscle needing attention with a bit of creative positioning of your body. Try not to stave off working on the very tender spots. When you come across them, linger for 10 to 30 seconds.

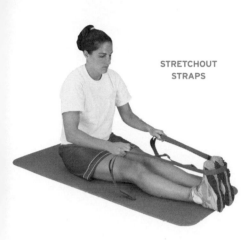

STRETCHOUT
STRAPS

STRETCHOUT STRAPS

THE FUNCTION Using these straps with certain stretches, especially those for the legs, will give you extra leverage and mobility. While lying on your back, loop one end around your foot while holding the other end in your hand(s) and pull your fully extended leg toward you until the sensation of the stretch makes you feel like you want to bend your knee, but don't have to. Hold the stretch for 10 to 30 seconds. Ask a trainer to show you a couple of stretching ideas with the straps.

SEATED STRETCH MACHINE

THE FUNCTION This funky stool-like apparatus enables you to stretch almost all muscle groups. It is very easy to use, and clear directions for each stretch are labeled on the machine.

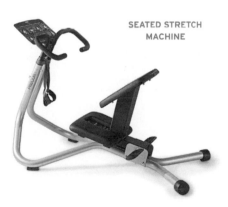

SEATED STRETCH
MACHINE

THE QUICK START

6

WE BEGIN this chapter with "The Essentials." The Essentials are 13
exercises to be done on strength training equipment, for the most part.
One of the exercises requires no equipment at all, and another, the use
of a Physio Ball. No. 9 is a three-part exercise, and No. 13 has two parts.
All of these exercises should be learned straight away. Together they
will give you a balanced, full-body workout and are an excellent initiation to your new fit life. Learn the mechanics of these moves, and try
them in the Time-Less Sample Workouts we have designed for you.
(You'll find the "Time-Less Samplers" later on in this chapter.) These
workouts will take you anywhere from 10 to 30 minutes and use only
exercises in "The Essentials."

Once you are well situated with the exercises in The Essentials, as
they are described, venture off into new territory. Learn to use other
machines and free weights targeting the same muscle groups and
interchange them at will.

Remember that the cardinal rule with working out is a sense of symmetry. Your master workout plan should always unite all different types of training (resistance, cardiovascular, core strength, balance, stability, flexibility, and stretching). Your resistance training should judiciously work all sides of your body. For example, be sure to work your chest as well as your back, your lower body as well as your upper body.

THE ESSENTIALS

1. Basic Smith Machine Squat
2. Basic Smith Machine Lunge
3. Smith Machine Straight Arm Plank with Hip Extension
4. Smith Machine Incline Push-Up
5. Smith Machine Modified Pull-Up
6. Seated Row Machine
7. Chest Press Machine
8. Shoulder Press Machine
9. Triple Hammy Whammy
10. Lat Pull-Down Machine
11. Lateral Raise Machine
12. Leg Press Machine
13. Planks (Front and Side)

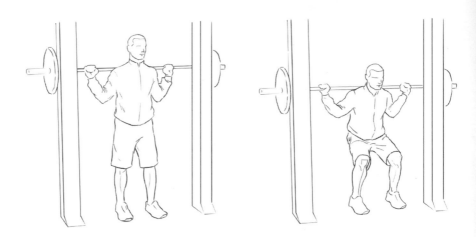

BASIC SMITH MACHINE SQUAT

THE SETUP Position the bar a few inches lower than shoulder height. With the bar resting across your back, just above your shoulder blades, lift and unhook the bar. Your feet should be a full step in front of the bar, hip to shoulder width apart, with toes pointing directly forward.

THE MOVE Slowly bend your knees up to a 90-degree angle and sit your hips back as if you were about to have a seat in a chair. Your weight should be directly over your ankles. Pause briefly at the lowest point before pushing your feet evenly into the floor and your hips forward to return to starting position. Repeat this move for the allotted repetitions with little or no pause at the top of the exercise.

CLUES (THESE CLUES ALSO APPLY TO DOING LUNGES):

1. Be attentive to the position of your knees. They should always be in line with your toes and never extend beyond them.

2. Draw your shoulder blades down and into your back. When this is done correctly, your chest should feel a bit like it is puffed up and proud, and lifted toward the ceiling.

3. Brace your core. (For more details on core bracing, refer back to page 76.)

4. Take a deep breath as you lower into the squat. Exhale with some vigor as you push your way through the toughest part of the squat.

5. Keep your chin lifted off your chest and your focus forward.

BASIC SMITH MACHINE LUNGE

THE SETUP Set yourself up as if you were doing a squat on the Smith machine. Take one big step back so that your feet are staggered.

THE MOVE Keeping your upper body upright, slowly bend your front knee up to a 90-degree angle. As you do this, lower the back knee directly toward the floor as if you were going to kneel down on it. You should feel most of your weight over the ankle of the front foot. Drive your front foot into the floor to return to starting position.

CLUES

See squat clues. They are the same.

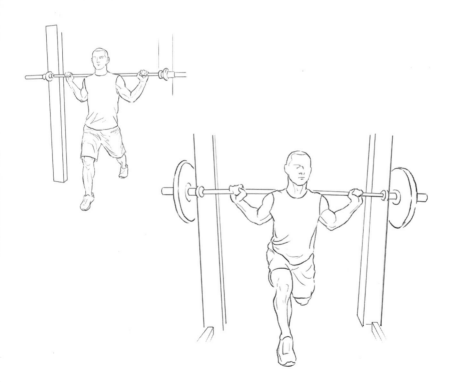

SMITH MACHINE STRAIGHT ARM PLANK WITH HIP EXTENSION

THE SETUP Set the bar at about chest height. (The higher you set the bar, the easier this exercise becomes. The lower you set it, the more difficult it becomes.) Firmly grasp the bar with your hands with an overhand grip, shoulder width apart or wider. Walk both feet back until your body is on an angle and in a strong straight line from head to toe. You should be on the balls of your feet.

THE MOVE Hold this straight arm plank position. Keeping your legs straight and your entire body in one straight line from head to toe, lift one foot toward the ceiling. Hold for a moment before returning to starting position. Repeat on the same side or alternate from side to side.

CLUES

1. Draw your shoulder blades down and into your back. When this is done correctly, your chest should feel a bit like it is puffed up and proud.

2. Brace your core. (For more details on core bracing, refer back to page 76.)

3. Keep your chin lifted off your chest and your focus on the floor in front of you.

4. Beware of letting your hips sag as you lift your foot off the floor.

5. Be sure to keep your hips squared off to the floor throughout the move.

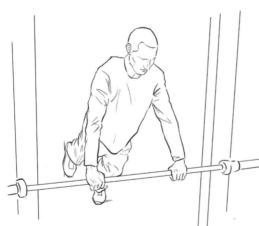

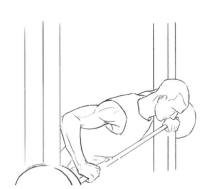

SMITH MACHINE INCLINE PUSH-UP

THE SETUP Set the bar at about chest height. (The higher you set the bar, the easier this exercise becomes. The lower you set it, the more difficult it becomes.) Firmly grasp the bar with your hands with an overhand grip, shoulder width apart or wider. Walk both feet back until your body is on an angle and in a strong straight line from head to toe. You should be on the balls of your feet.

THE MOVE Keeping your body in a strong straight planklike position, bend your elbows and lower your chest toward the bar. Your elbows should be at a 90-degree angle and the middle of your chest above the bar. Push into the bar with force until your arms are fully extended with elbows unlocked.

CLUES

1. Draw your shoulder blades down and into your back. When this is done correctly, your chest should feel a bit like it is puffed up and proud, and lifted toward the ceiling.

2. Brace your core. (For more details on core bracing, refer back to page 76.)

3. Take a deep breath as you lower your chest toward the bar. Exhale with some vigor as you push your body away from it.

4. Keep your chin lifted off your chest and your focus on the floor in front of you.

SMITH MACHINE MODIFIED PULL-UP

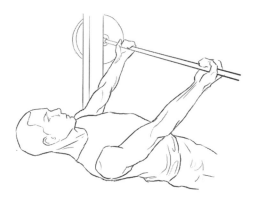

THE SETUP Set the bar at about chest height, higher to decrease difficulty and lower to increase difficulty. Grasp the bar with an underhand grip approximately shoulder width apart and walk your feet forward until you are hanging from the bar with your hands. Keep your body in a strong, straight line from head to toe.

THE MOVE Firmly pull your chest to the bar. Hold briefly before slowly lowering your body back down to starting position.

CLUES

1. As you pull your body up, keep your chin lifted off your chest.

2. Imagine driving your elbows down and back as you lift your chest to the bar. You should feel like you are puffing out your chest.

3. Brace your core. (For more details on core bracing, refer back to page 76.)

4. Exhale as you pull your body up and inhale as you lower it down.

5. To make the exercise a bit easier, keep your knees slightly bent and your feet closer to the bar.

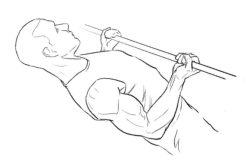

SEATED ROW MACHINE

THE SETUP Have a seat; if the machine you are using has foot stops, place your feet on them. Set the seat high enough so that the chest pad is at the middle of your chest. Adjust the distance of the chest pad so that you can just reach the handles. Grasp the handles on the rowing machine. Sit upright.

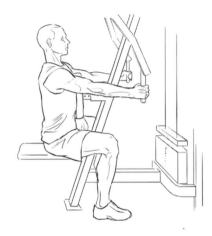

THE MOVE Sit tall and drive your elbows back toward your body. As you pull, squeeze your shoulder blades together. Hold briefly before slowly returning to starting position. Be sure your chest maintains contact with the chest pad as you pull the handles toward your body.

CLUES

1. Exhale as you pull and inhale as you return to starting position.

2. Draw your shoulder blades down and into your back. When this is done correctly, your chest should feel a bit like it is puffed up and proud, and lifted toward the ceiling.

3. Brace your core. (For more details on core bracing, refer back to page 76.)

4. As you pull, continue to sit upright and resist the urge to lean back.

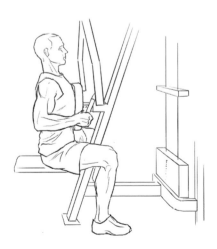

CHEST PRESS MACHINE

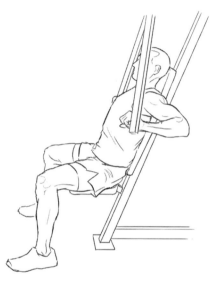

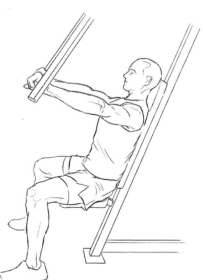

THE SETUP Set the seat so that if there were a line from one handle to the other, it would cross the middle of your chest. Sit back and let your head and back rest against the support. If the machine you are using has a foot bar, push it forward until you can comfortably grasp the handles. Grasp the handles firmly with strong, straight wrists. Your elbows should be at about a 90-degree angle. Keep your elbows up so that they are about the same height as the handles.

THE MOVE Drive the bar away from you until your arms are fully extended, with elbows unlocked. Slowly return to starting position where your elbows are bent about 90 degrees.

CLUES

1. Imagine you are pushing your back through the back support as you drive the bar away from you. Be careful not to round your back.

2. Exhale as you push and inhale as you lower back to starting position.

SHOULDER PRESS MACHINE

THE SETUP Set the seat height so that the handles are just above shoulder height when seated. Have a seat with your hips, back, and head resting firmly against the back support. Grasp the handles securely with your palms facing forward, with strong, straight wrists.

THE MOVE Push the handles toward the ceiling until your arms are fully extended, with elbows unlocked. Slowly lower to starting position.

CLUES

1. Exhale as you push up and inhale as you lower the handles.

2. As you press up, draw your shoulder blades down and into your back. When this is done correctly, your neck should feel long and your chest should feel a bit like it is puffed up, proud, and lifted toward the ceiling.

3. Brace your core. (For more details on core bracing, refer back to page 76.)

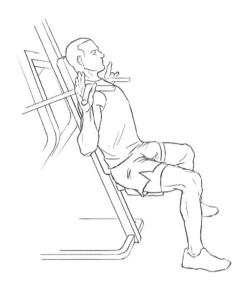

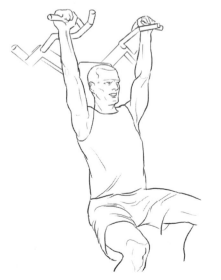

TRIPLE HAMMY WHAMMY

(This is a three-part exercise we learned from Juan Carlos Santana, M.Ed., CSCS, one of the top trainers in the United States. It requires the use of a Physio Ball.)

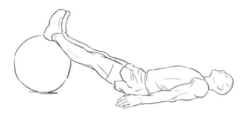

Part I

THE SETUP Lie on your back with your arms at your sides and your heels resting on top of the Physio Ball. Your toes should be facing the ceiling and your legs fully extended.

THE MOVE Drive your heels into the Physio Ball as you push your hips toward the ceiling until you are in a bridgelike position. Your heels, hips, and shoulders should create a strong straight line. Hold briefly before lowering your hips back to the floor. Lightly touch your rear end to the floor. Repeat 8 to 15 times before moving onto Part II of this exercise.

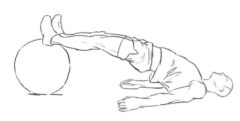

Part II

THE SETUP Continue lying on your back with your arms at your sides. Raise your hips to a bridge-like position with your knees, hips, and shoulders in a straight line.

THE MOVE Pull your heels in toward your rear end as far as you can. Push your heels back out away from you, back to the bridge position. Throughout this move, keep your hips as high off the ground as possible. Repeat 8 to 15 times before moving on to Part III of this exercise.

Part III

THE SETUP Roll the Physio Ball away from you until you can just reach it with the balls of your feet with your legs fully extended.

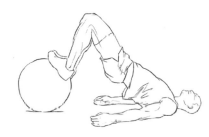

THE MOVE Push the balls of your feet into the Physio Ball as you push your hips toward the ceiling until you are in a bridge position. Hold briefly before lowering your hips toward the floor. Lightly touch the floor with your rear end, and repeat 8 to 15 times.

Start this exercise by doing eight reps per part, one to three times. Add an additional rep a week until you've reached 15. If you are feeling ambitious, you can progress once again from 8 to 15 reps using one foot at a time.

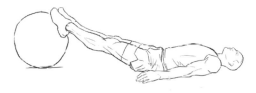

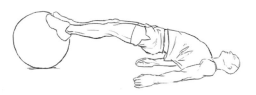

LAT PULL-DOWN MACHINE

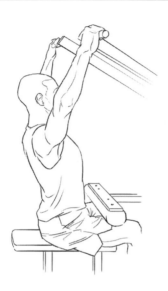

THE SETUP Adjust the seat so that your legs are firmly secured under the leg support and when your arms are fully extended the handles are just out of reach. If there is a chest pad on the machine you are using, it should be in the middle of your chest. Grasp the handles securely. Lock your shoulder blades down and into your back. When this is done correctly, your neck should feel long and your chest should feel a bit like it is puffed up, proud, and lifted toward the ceiling.

THE MOVE Drive your elbows down and back toward your body. Hold for a moment before returning to starting position.

CLUES

1. The movement should be slow and controlled.
2. Keep your chest lifted throughout the movement.

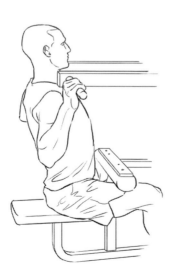

LATERAL RAISE MACHINE

THE SETUP Set the seat height so that when you are sitting on the machine your shoulders are aligned with its pivots. Sit facing the machine with the outside of your forearms on the pads and lightly grasp the handles.

THE MOVE Raise your elbows away from your body to shoulder height. Hold for a moment and slowly return to starting position.

CLUES

1. The pads should not be sliding around on your arms during the exercise. If they are, you probably need to adjust your seat.

2. Keep your shoulder blades down and into your back. Your chest should be lifted and feel like it is puffing out. Your neck will feel long.

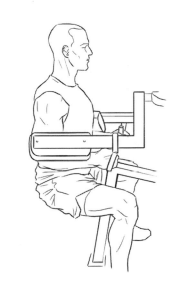

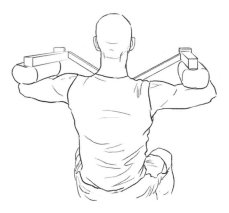

LEG PRESS MACHINE

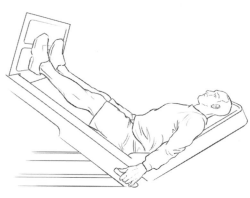

THE SETUP Sit in the machine with your hips, back, shoulders, and head resting against the back rest. Place your feet hip to shoulder width apart on the upper-middle part of the platform with your toes pointing straight up. Grasp the handles securely and comfortably.

THE MOVE Brace your core and roll your shoulder blades down and back. Press the platform away from you until your legs are fully extended, but your knees unlocked. Disengage the safety mechanism and slowly bend your knees up to 90 degrees. You should feel most of the weight on your heels and middle of your feet. Push back to starting position.

CLUES

1. Exhale as you push, inhale as you bend your knees.

2. Keep your knees lined up with your big and second toes throughout the move.

3. Keep your heels on the platform.

4. Do not tuck your pelvis throughout this exercise.

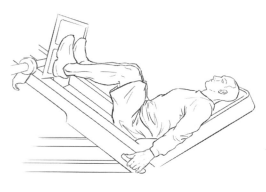

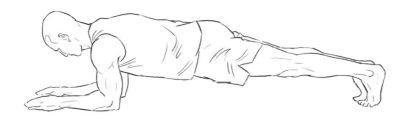

PLANKS: FRONT PLANK

THE SETUP Begin with your elbows and knees on the floor. Your elbows should be directly under your shoulders. Your body should be in a straight line from your head to your knees.

THE MOVE Brace your core. Push your toes into the floor as you lift your knees so that your body is in a straight "planklike" line from your head to your toes. Engage all the muscles of your body from head to toe. Hold this position for the allotted amount of time.

CLUES

1. Strive to keep your hips from sagging toward the floor or piking up toward the ceiling.

2. To make the move easier, do it from your knees.

3. To start, try to hold the plank position for 20 seconds. As you become stronger, increase the amount of time up to 60 seconds or longer.

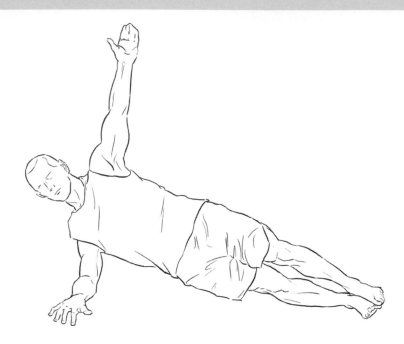

PLANKS: SIDE PLANK

THE SETUP Begin lying on your side with your elbow on the floor directly under your shoulder. Your forearm should be on the floor at a right angle to your body, with your palms facing down. Your hips should be perfectly perpendicular to the floor and your feet should be stacked one on top of the other.

THE MOVE Push your elbow and lower foot into the floor to lift your hips toward the ceiling until your body is in a straight "planklike" line from head to foot. Engage of the muscles of your body from head to toe. Hold this position for the allotted amount of time.

CLUES

1. Strive to keep your hips from sagging toward the floor.

2. To make the move easier, either split your legs so that the top leg is in front of the lower leg, or do it from your knees by bending your knees to a 90-degree angle.

3. To start, try to hold the plank position for 20 seconds. As you become stronger, increase the amount of time up to 60 seconds or longer.

4. Don't forget to work both sides evenly.

IDEAS FOR A WARM-UP

We've already discussed how important it is to warm up before your workout, and here we are telling you again (repetition is the secret to retention). A warm-up primes you for the workout to come by circulating blood freely through your muscles and raising your body temperature. Your body and mind are set into the position and feeling of readiness. A light sweat and a focused mental state should characterize the end of your warm-up. Some warm-up suggestions are:

1. Spend 5 to 10 minutes doing a low-intensity warm-up on any of the cardio equipment at your gym—a brisk walk or light jog on the treadmill and a leisurely ride on a stationary bike are terrific ways to get your muscles ready for the work ahead of them.

2. Begin with a 10- to 15-minute core-specific workout.

3. Warming up for resistance training can be as simple as slowly waking the muscle group you are getting ready to train with a taste test. Do this by beginning each new exercise with a full set using light weights.

TIME-LESS SAMPLE WORKOUTS

So you've learned the mechanics behind the "Essential" moves. To help send you off without further hesitation, we've put together three very easy-to-follow workouts using only the exercises in "The Essentials."

THE SMITH MACHINE WORKOUT

THE HIGHLIGHT Full Body

SETS Up to three

REPS 12 to 15

TIME Doing one set of each exercise will take approximately 5 to 8 minutes. Doing three sets will take approximately 15 to 24 minutes.

THE PROTOCOL It's all about you and the Smith machine with this workout. You only need this one piece of equipment—it's as simple as that. Complete the full number of sets for each exercise before moving on to the next. Recover for 30 to 60 seconds in between sets, depending on how hard the set is.

THE MOVES

1

Smith Machine Straight Arm
Plank with Hip Extension
(12 to 15 reps per side)

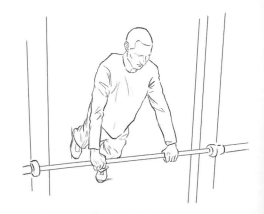

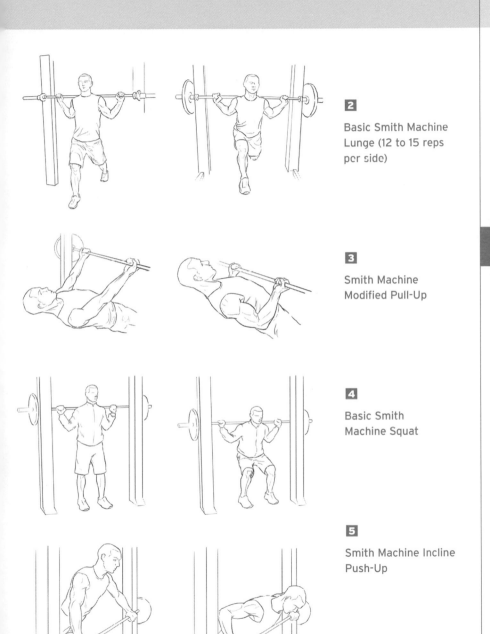

2

Basic Smith Machine Lunge (12 to 15 reps per side)

3

Smith Machine Modified Pull-Up

4

Basic Smith Machine Squat

5

Smith Machine Incline Push-Up

THE EQUALIZER CIRCUIT

THE HIGHLIGHT Full Body with Cardio Blast

SETS Complete circuit one to three times

REPS 12 to 15

TIME Doing one set of each exercise will take approximately 15 minutes. Doing three sets will take approximately 45 minutes.

THE PROTOCOL You'll need the assistance of a few different machines for this workout. Move from one exercise to the next through the full circuit. The cardio blasts should last three minutes. We suggest jumping rope, but feel free to exchange that with jumping jacks, riding a stationary bike, or running on the treadmill. It is up to you. Ideally, your recovery should be just enough time to move on to the next machine and set up, approximately 30 seconds.

THE MOVES

1

Basic Smith Machine Squat

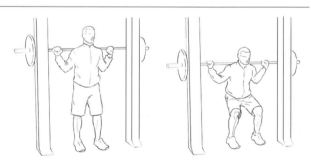

2

Chest Press

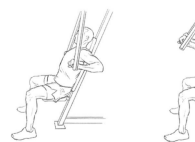

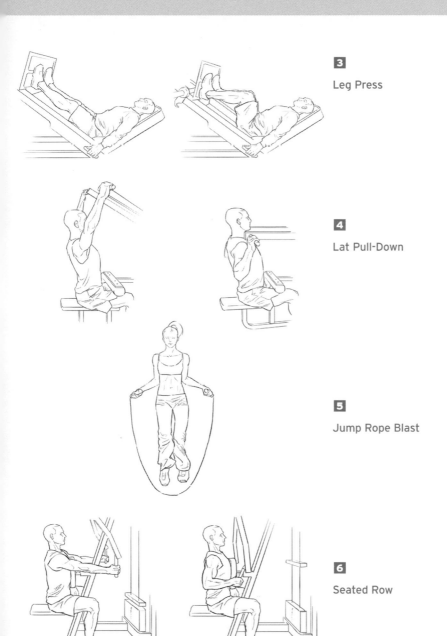

3

Leg Press

4

Lat Pull-Down

5

Jump Rope Blast

6

Seated Row

7

Shoulder Press

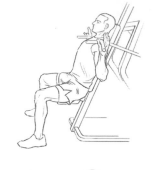
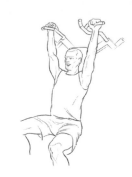

8

Smith Machine Straight Arm Plank with Hip Extension (12 to 15 reps per side)

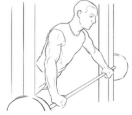
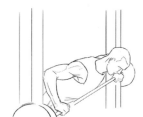

9

Lateral Raise

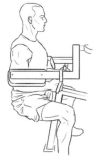
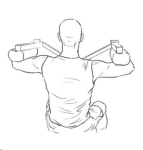

10

Jump Rope Blast

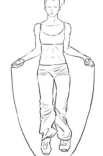

THE QUICK START

THE NUTS AND BOLTS WORKOUT

THE HIGHLIGHT Full Body

SETS Up to three

REPS 12 to 15

TIME Doing one set of each exercise will take approximately 10 minutes. Doing three sets will take approximately 30 minutes.

THE PROTOCOL You'll need the assistance of a few different machines for this workout. Complete the full number of sets for each exercise before moving on to the next. For the first exercises (front and side planks) hold each position for 20 to 60 seconds. The next exercise, the Triple Hammy Whammy, you will recall from "The Essentials," is a devil of an exercise. Start off doing eight reps and see how you feel at the end. Add an additional rep or two to make the circuit more challenging as you become stronger.

THE MOVES

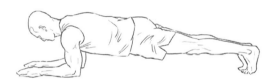

Front Plank

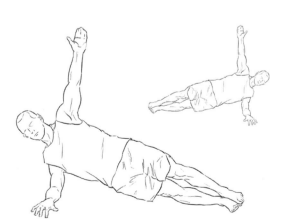

Side Plank

Opposite Side Plank

Triple Hammy Whammy

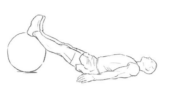

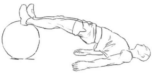

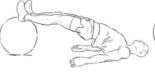

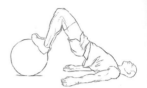

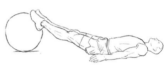

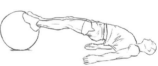

Basic Smith Machine Lunge (12 to 15 reps each side)

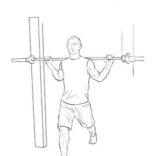

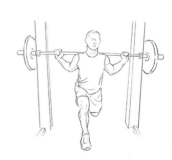

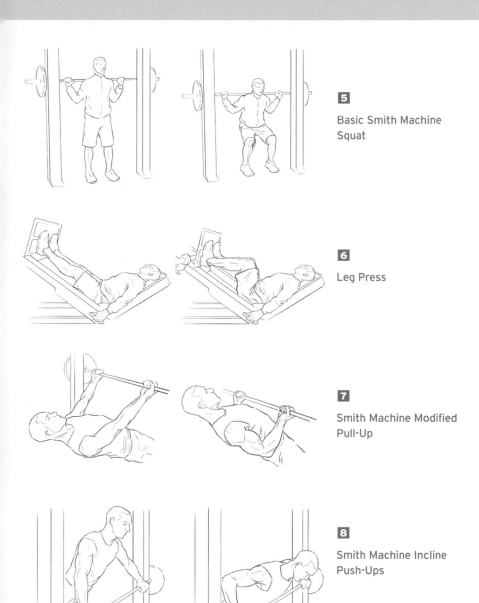

5

Basic Smith Machine Squat

6

Leg Press

7

Smith Machine Modified Pull-Up

8

Smith Machine Incline Push-Ups

9

Shoulder Press

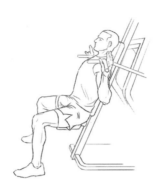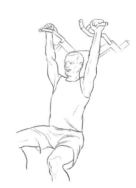

10

Lateral Raise

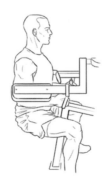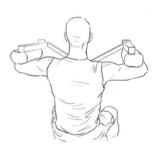

TRAINING DAYS

How often should I exercise? Here are some general guidelines.

BEGINNER

As a fitness fledgling, we recommend starting with a two- to three-day-a-week commitment in order to reap rewards without wiping yourself out. Always allow yourself at least one day of rest in between training days. Progression to the next level will be natural. When you're ready for more, your current workouts won't feel as challenging as they once felt.

INTERMEDIATE

As you move on in your training and become more conditioned, you'll need more challenging workouts in order to continue your progress. Eventually, you will be ready to trade a few rest days for additional training days. At this point, you can add one to two extra training days to your workout week because your body won't need as much rest time to recover. However, you will need to become more creative with your training approach. For example, you can alternate harder days with easier days and cardio training with strength training throughout the week. This is a good time to speak with a trainer about creating the right schedule for you and your specific goals.

ADVANCED

At this juncture, training will be deeply embedded in your life and you may want to up the training ante to six days a week. Your body of knowledge is probably pretty sophisticated by now, so you won't need our help planning and organizing your workout schedule. You're ready to fly solo!

EXAMPLES OF TRAINING DAY GAME PLANS

	Sunday	Monday	Tuesday	Wednesday	Thursday	Friday	Saturday
BEGINNER 2 Days a Week	Rest	TRAIN	Rest	Rest	Rest	TRAIN	Rest
BEGINNER 3 Days a Week	Rest	TRAIN	Rest	TRAIN	Rest	TRAIN	Rest
INTERMEDIATE 4 Days a Week	Rest	TRAIN	TRAIN	Rest	TRAIN	Rest	TRAIN
INTERMEDIATE 5 Days a Week	Rest	TRAIN	TRAIN	Rest	TRAIN	TRAIN	TRAIN

TROUBLE SPOT STRETCHES

Here are a few remedies for relieving the most common tight spots. Don't feel limited to the stretches we are offering. You're free to do any type of stretch you prefer as long as you, or the person assisting you in the stretch, know what you're doing. Injuries caused by stretching gone wrong are not as uncommon as you may think, so proceed with caution.

THE LOWDOWN

STRETCHING INSIGHT

Did you know that when we stretch, we are actually causing a minute amount of damage to our muscles? Not to worry; it's amazing how quickly such damage repairs itself—just like magic. We learned this from our aforementioned friend and author of *Full Body Flexibility*, Jay Blahnik. The best time to stretch is after a workout, when all the muscles in your body are warm and supple. Theoretically, you are at greater risk of injury otherwise.

THE TIGHT SPOT: HAMSTRINGS

THE PRESCRIPTION Single Leg Forward Bend

THE DIRECTIONS Begin standing with most of your body weight on one leg and that knee unlocked. Drive the heel of the non-weight-bearing leg toward the ceiling, hinging at the hips, until you feel the stretch in the hamstring of the standing leg. Keep your arms at your sides or like wings reaching out to the sides. Your body will be in one straight line from your head to the heel of the back leg. Hold for 15 to 45 seconds. If balance is an issue, lightly hold on to something for support.

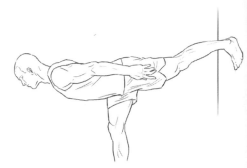

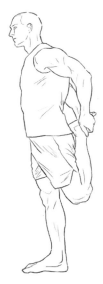

THE TIGHT SPOT: QUADRICEPS

THE PRESCRIPTION Standing Quadriceps Stretch

THE DIRECTIONS Begin standing with most of your body weight on one leg and knee unlocked. Grasp the foot of the non-weight-bearing leg in your hand and pull your heel toward the gluteals until you feel a stretch in your quadriceps. For a deeper stretch, push the heel into your gluteals further and keep your knees aligned. Hold for 15 to 45 seconds. If balance is an issue, lightly hold on to something for support.

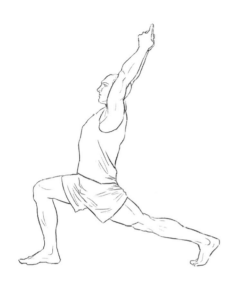

THE TIGHT SPOT: HIP FLEXOR

THE PRESCRIPTION Deep Lunge

THE DIRECTIONS In a deep lunge push through the hip as you lift through the chest and extend your arms to the ceiling until you feel the stretch at the top of the back leg into the lower region of the abdominals. Hold for 15 to 45 seconds.

THE TIGHT SPOT: GLUTEALS

THE PRESCRIPTION Standing Ankle to Knee Stretch

THE DIRECTIONS Begin standing with most of your body weight on one leg and knee unlocked. Bring the ankle of the non-weight-bearing leg across the opposite knee. Keeping the back flat, bend your standing leg and push your hips back as you lunge forward until you feel the stretch in the gluteals of the crossed leg. Extend your arms out in front of you for counterbalance. Hold for 15 to 45 seconds. If you're having trouble maintaining your balance, hold on to something for support or try assuming the stretch position while seated.

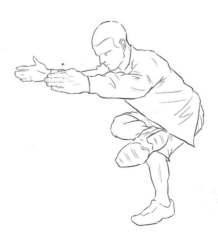

213

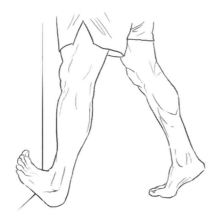

THE TIGHT SPOT: CALVES

THE PRESCRIPTION Calf Stretch

THE DIRECTIONS Begin standing in front of a wall with the ball of one foot on the wall and the heel of that foot on the floor. With your legs straight, push your hips in toward the wall until you feel a sufficient stretch in your calf. Keep a straight line from the top of your head, down to your heel. Hold for 15 to 45 seconds.

THE TIGHT SPOT: CHEST

THE PRESCRIPTION Chest Stretch

THE DIRECTIONS Extend both elbows directly out to the sides with your fingertips lightly touching the back of your head. Reach back with both elbows squeezing your shoulder blades together. You should feel the stretch through your chest and front of your shoulders. Imagine trying to touch your elbows behind your back. Keep your neck long. Hold for a few seconds, release, and repeat 10 to 15 times.

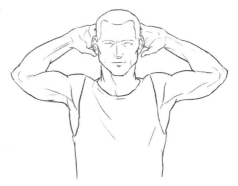

THE TIGHT SPOT: BACK

THE PRESCRIPTION Standing Lat Stretch

THE DIRECTIONS Begin in a standing position, holding both arms out in front of your body with fingers interlocked. Sit back into a squat as you curl your torso into a curved C-shape while pulling your arms to one side. You should feel the stretch down the side of your back. Hold for 15 to 45 seconds and repeat on the opposite side.

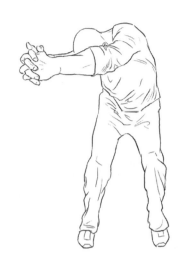

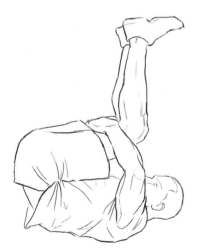

THE TIGHT SPOT: LOWER BACK

THE PRESCRIPTION Lower Back Roll

THE DIRECTIONS Lie on your back locking your arms underneath your knees. Pull your knees toward you until your hips and lower back roll off the floor. Hold for a moment, release, and repeat. You can also try rolling your hips in a circular motion.

THE CODE OF
GYM CONDUCT

7

HAVE YOUR EFFORTS to locate any of Emily Post's books of etiquette for appropriate gym behavior been successful? Highly doubtful! As we have mentioned throughout this book, the gym world is unique, and such information is not widely distributed.

Our closing topic of discussion, the code of gym conduct, is unlike the rest of this book in that it will not directly help you to attain a fitter, stronger, or healthier body. It will, however, give you an idea of what to wear, how to act, and what to bring with you to the gym. You will then look and act the part of an experienced, long-standing gym member. As a bonus, you can bet on having an open-armed welcome by both gym management and fellow members.

DRESS CODE

Engaging in activities that may require you to assume some curious or ostensibly compromising positions is fairly commonplace at the gym, so we'll say a few words on the topic of dress codes. No, working out shouldn't be mistaken for a fashion show and you won't be judged on whether or not you're dressed in line with the latest fashion frenzy. There are, however, a few intricacies about dressing appropriately for a workout that, lacking any previous experience, you aren't likely to know.

It's important to dress for the occasion. You wouldn't wear a wedding dress to a barbeque, would you? You should plan on investing a bit in workout clothing, if for nothing more than inspiration. Workout clothing will get you in the right mind-set. Don't wear your new pair of jeans to the gym and assume they'll work just because they are stretchy.

THE UNDERGARMENTS

Adequately covering, stretchy, and supportive undergarments are crucial. You may be bending down or waving your legs in the air at some point during your workout. If you're sporting loose-fitting shorts, be sure to wear some type of tight keep-it-together shorts underneath them. Male or female, you really don't want any uncouth peek-a-boo action going on every time you make a move. If you're a man and wear a jockstrap, make sure it doesn't make an appearance anywhere outside the locker room.

For the ladies, panty lines are not attractive in any situation. They won't flatter your gluteus maximus, and will accentu-ate any surplus padding you may have around that area. Go for thongs or boy shorts that won't cut into your cheeks. Many workout shorts and pants are designed to free you from the necessity of having to wear additional undergarments at all.

Also for the ladies: be sure to wear a figure-hugging sports bra, even if you wear a shirt over it. Test your sports bras before you wear them to the gym. Jump around. Do cartwheels. Shake rigorously. Be sure your sports bra doesn't unravel, unbutton, or untie. If anything comes undone or pops out—yes, we've seen this happen—you need to find a better sports bra.

THE FIT

Do not be ashamed of your figure. You're at the gym and you should be proud. Regardless of how much gym-related experience you have tucked under your belt, remember that your peers at the gym all share the same goal as you—to become healthier and more physically fit. Don't wear clothing that is too big for you in an attempt to hide your figure flaws—overly baggy shirts and pants may actually be a hazard. Extra fabric can get caught on equipment and can also wrap itself around you as you work out, restricting your movements and causing discomfort. On the other side of the coin, avoid wearing anything that is too tight and cuts off your circulation.

Don't be ashamed of your figure. If you have great legs, show them off. Wear shorts. Wear leggings that show off the contours of your legs. If you have ripped abs, put them out on display. You'll inspire others around you and yourself.

Beware of workout shorts or shirts in pale or pastel colors. They accentuate all the areas that are damp with sweat by

THE LOWDOWN

CLANDESTINE COLORS

Black is a secret weapon. You've heard it a million times because it is quite true. Black is masking and slimming. It is also non-attention-grabbing and won't become transparent when wet.

becoming see-through or by turning a very contrasting shade. Well-lined and high-tech fabrics may be the exception to the rule.

Horizontal stripes will make you look wider. Vertical stripes will make you look longer. Too many stripes of any sort may make you and anyone looking at you dizzy.

FABRIC INFO AND PROPER CARE

Snug-fitting workout gear made from stretchy, breathable fabric is great. Although there are many high-tech fabrics to choose from, some of our favorites include: Lycra, Supplex, Coolmax, and Dri-FIT (by Nike). Workout clothes made out of these materials allow you to move freely and comfortably. Coolmax and Dri-FIT work in a vacuumlike fashion by pulling moisture away from your body to the surface layer of the garment, allowing it to evaporate and dry quickly. These fibers will allow you to move without restraint, while keeping you drier and cooler throughout your workout.

Toss your sweaty workout clothes into the washing machine as soon as possible. Wash high-tech fabrics in cold water and then dry them on low heat or, better yet, hang them up to dry. If you can't do a load of laundry after every workout, rinse

THE LOWDOWN

BAG IT

Bring your sweaty clothing home to be laundered in a plastic bag to avoid contaminating everything else in your gym bag, or the bag itself. If you don't do this, eventually your bag will be permanently soiled by a combination of undesirable body odors and wet marks.

and soak the just-worn outfit in laundry detergent to prolong the life of the fabric. Keep in mind that no matter how well you take care of your gear, you'll probably need to replace the clothing after three to six months of use. Make sure to consider this when figuring out how much to spend on fitness clothing.

INSIDER INFO

Beware of sports bras with cumbersome embellishments. Heavy hardware, such as zippers and buttons, and even simple decorative knots can sometimes get in your way. While they may look pretty and even feel comfortable when you're standing still, such decorations often rub against your skin while you work out and cause irritations or rashes. Make it a point to be as comfortable as possible and avoid clothing that will interfere with your workout. Having to tug, pull up, pull down, or adjust your clothing in any way is definitely a disturbance.

Put on a clean set of workout clothes each time you hit the gym. If there's even a hint of a sour odor caused by old sweat hidden in the fibers of your clothing, it will be accentuated by the heat and additional moisture expelled during your next workout. You should always expect to break a sweat during your training session. So, showing up at the gym wearing dirty, foulsmelling gear that you know is just going to get smellier over the course of your workout is downright offensive. Don't torture yourself and everyone around you.

Ladies: There's no need to put on makeup before heading to the gym. The combination of sweat and makeup is unsightly, and although we're not dermatologists, we feel it's pretty safe to assume that this isn't the best way to treat your pores.

The gym is not the place to show off your bling, so limit the amount of jewelry you wear. There are several reasons for this.

- **Your jewels may get caught on the equipment and either break or end up hurting you.**

- **Because (hopefully) you'll be moving around a lot, there's a pretty good possibility that you'll lose whatever jewelry you're wearing.**

- **It's an invitation for theft.**

FOOTWEAR

All gyms require that you wear some type of closed-toe training shoe. The reason for this is simple—exposed toes are not safe in a gym. If a weight is accidentally dropped on your bare foot, you can expect to feel quite a bit of pain. Closed-toe shoes are the way to go and unprotected feet are a lawsuit waiting to happen—trust us.

The many different types of training shoes on the market are designed with specific activities in mind. In order to ensure the best success when engaging in different kinds of activities at the gym, see our Footwear-Activity Match-Up chart below.

FOOTWEAR-ACTIVITY MATCH-UP

ACTIVITY	SHOE
Running (Outdoors, Track, or Treadmill)	**Running shoe**
Cardiovascular Training on Equipment (Stationary Bike, Rowing Machine, Stepper, and so on.)	**Any training shoe**
Aerobic Classes (Step, Hi-Low, Dance, BOSU, Urban Rebounding, Kickboxing, Jump Rope, and so on.)	**Any type of training shoe is acceptable,** but a cross-training shoe offering a wide base and plenty of lateral support works best.
Indoor Cycling Class	**Cycling shoe.** Ask your gym what type of clips their bikes are fitted with so that you can purchase the appropriate pair of shoes. All indoor cycling classes will be able to accommodate trainers as well.
Aqua Class	**Water shoes**
Yoga, Pilates	**Bare feet**
Weight Training (on training floor)	**Any training shoe**

THE FUNDAMENTAL GYM BAG CHECKLIST

Take a little time to consider which of the following items you need to include in your gym bag.

Gym membership/access/ID card

Combination lock (It can be a pain to carry around the key to your lock.)

Bottle of water or sports drink

Workout clothes

Extra T-shirt

Socks

Sneakers

Hair tie (if you have long hair)

Special equipment (cycling shoes, yoga mat)

Training gloves

Walkman, portable CD player, or iPod/portable MP3 player

Heart-rate monitor

Deodorant

Towel (if not provided by your gym)

Rubber slippers or flip-flops

Shower supplies (shampoo, soap, and so on), if not provided by your gym

Hairbrush/hair dryer (dryers will sometimes be provided by your gym)

Toothbrush/toothpaste/mouthwash

Empty plastic bag (for sweaty clothing)

Emergency contact/medical information

Training workbook or log

Gym Survival Guide

It's a good idea to keep a permanent locker at the gym if you're planning to go from the gym directly to the office, or vice versa. Doing so can save you the hassle of lugging everything back and forth, and you can store most of the contents of your gym bag in your locker. You should also consider keeping a complete set of extra workout clothes in your locker, along with any other special equipment you may have—yoga mat, cycling shoes, and the like.

THE LOWDOWN
SAVE YOUR HANDS
Invest in a pair of training gloves. They'll allow you to focus on your training and not the discomfort in your hands.

BEHAVE YOURSELF

During the majority of our day-to-day interactions with others, we happily abide by the rules of etiquette painstakingly drilled into us by our parents. Such rules of conduct are often so deeply ingrained in us that we are no longer conscious of them. At the gym, however, these rules are sometimes cast aside and counteretiquette surfaces in their place. In all fairness, it must be noted that the gym is a world completely unlike the one our parents trained us for, and so there are some behavioral intricacies specific to the gym environment that require clarification. Some of the rules listed below may seem obvious, but because they are broken on a regular basis, we felt they were worth mentioning.

GENERAL RULES OF GYM ETIQUETTE

Do not stink. Because you know you're going to sweat during your workout doesn't mean it's okay to skip on the shower before you hit the gym. Also, don't try to get more than one wear out of your gym clothes before washing them. Just because the sweat has dried up doesn't mean the clothes are clean.

No perfume, please. If you didn't bathe before going to the gym, don't try to mask your body odor with strong-scented perfumes. In fact, refrain from wearing any perfume at all. This can be as offensives, if not more offensive than, natural body odor in the gym.

Brush your teeth. Bad breath, whether the result of a sour stomach or the garlic bread you had with lunch, is bad news. Bad breath in a group fitness class packed with many other people, all breathing heavily, has the potential to ruin the workout experience for everyone.

No spitting in the water fountains. That's just disgusting.

Don't leave a sweaty piece of equipment behind for the next person. Wipe it off with a towel and/or any disinfectant spray supplied by the gym.

THE CODE OF GYM CONDUCT

Put your toys away after you're done playing with them. Don't leave the weights you just used scattered all over the gym floor for someone else to trip on or put away for you. If you're strong enough to use them, you're strong enough to carry them back to where they came from.

Gym equipment is not yours alone. Share, especially if the gym is crowded. If you see that there is someone waiting patiently for the piece of equipment you're using, consider letting him or her work in with you. This means that while you rest between sets, they work in their own set. Use this time productively. For example, try out an interim exercise that targets or stretches a different muscle group or work on your balance with a wobble board. Sharing also means that once you're finished with a piece of equipment, walk away. Do not linger on it while trying to figure out what you're going to do next.

Sharing also applies to cardio equipment, especially when the gym is crowded. Some gyms will set time limits on popular cardio machines during the busiest times of the day. Pay attention to them.

No one likes to be startled by sudden bursts of loud noise, especially while they're lifting heavy weights. Don't let equipment fall on the floor— it's not only annoying and disruptive, but also potentially dangerous.

No cell phones, Blackberries, walkie-talkies or anything of the sort in the gym. Here's the hidden danger: if you're on one of these gadgets and consumed in conversation, you're likely not paying attention to what you or anyone around you is doing. Also, you should be using your time at the gym to work out, not chat on your cell phone or send emails from your blackberry. There is a time and place for everything. Don't waste your time at the gym on the phone. Plus it is annoying.

Mind the way you sound in the gym. Normal sounds induced by big efforts are totally fine, but be conscious of how you express yourself. Vulgarities are unpleasant anywhere, including the gym.

When taking a group fitness class, think back to your school days. Don't carry on a conversation during class. It's not only disruptive, but you're also more likely to miss your instructor's next cue if you're not paying attention.

No headphones in class. If you really enjoy a particular instructor's class, but prefer to groove to a different beat, kindly offer to bring in music suggestions you think would work. The instructor will most likely appreciate this and try to work your tunes into the class.

Even if you're always on the same spin bike or in the same spot in a group fitness class, remember that you do not own the space. Don't get angry with other people who take "your spot."

It is great to be able to see yourself in the mirror while you're training or in a group fitness class in order to check yourself for proper form, but be conscious of your neighbors and don't monopolize the mirror space. Check to see that you're not blocking someone else's view if possible.

Be respectful of your neighbor's space and don't set up your equipment so that it is too close to anyone else's. Also look to see that you're not directly in front of anyone in a group fitness class.

STEAM ROOM COMMANDMENTS

The steam room is often a haven for misbehaving. There are a few especially offensive activities that should be avoided at all costs. We lay down the top three commandments below.

- Do not clip your finger or toenails.

- Do not de-fur any part of your body in the steam room.

- Last, but absolutely not least, the steam room is definitely not the appropriate place to re-ignite a romance gone cold (or the place for *any* activity of that nature).

GLOSSARY

Abduction Moving a body part away from the body's central axis. For example, when you perform a hip abduction, you move your legs away from an imaginary line that runs vertically through the center of your body.

Abs (abdominals) The abdominal muscles make up your body's midsection. This muscle group includes all of the following: the rectus abdominus, serratus, internal and external obliques, psoas, linea alba, linea similunaris, linea transversae, transversalis, and intercostals. The most visible abdominal muscle—the "six-pack" or rectus abdominus—extends from the bottom of your ribcage all the way to the hips; it controls the pelvic tilt and the flexion of the spine. The well-known "obliques" are composed of three separate muscle groups: the internal, transverse, and external obliques. These muscles are indispensable supporters of the vertebral column.

Active-isolated stretching This is an athletic stretching technique that involves activating the opposing muscle group to initiate the stretch for two seconds, releasing and repeating 10 times or so.

Adduction Moving a body part toward the body's central axis. For example, when you perform a hip adduction, you move your legs toward an imaginary line that runs vertically through the center of your body.

Aerobic Literally, this means "with oxygen." To exercise aerobically means to produce energy with oxygen. When we train aerobically, we train the body to become more efficient at using oxygen for energy.

Anaerobic Literally, this means "without oxygen." Anaerobic exercise, which often involves short, intense bursts of activity, uses up oxygen faster than the heart and lungs can produce it. Instead of using oxygen, the body turns to energy within the muscles to sustain the brief periods of intense exertion. Broadly speaking, this type of exercise is done in the form of interval training.

Asana Poses or postures in yoga.

Ballistic stretching Using the momentum of a moving part of the body to force it to stretch beyond its normal range of motion. The muscles are stretched using jerking or bouncing movements. Ballistic stretching is commonly frowned upon because it can lead to injury. Muscles are not given the opportunity to adjust and relax into the stretched position, causing them to react in the opposite manner and tighten up. An example of ballistic stretching: bending over and bouncing to try to touch your toes.

Biceps The biceps, or biceps brachii, make it possible for you to flex your elbows to bring your wrists toward your shoulders, and also allow you to rotate your forearms. Additionally, the biceps are supporting muscles for any pulling exercise targeting the muscles of the back.

Body fat The percentage of fat your body contains.

Burnout A term identifying the state of being bored with exercise. This is usually what happens as a result of consistently doing the same type of workout and/or not having adequate rest.

Cadence The timing of motion; for example, the speed of your pedaling if you are on a bicycle.

Calisthenics Resistance exercises using body weight only. For example, push-ups, jumping jacks, crunches, and basic squats.

Cardiovascular Involving the heart, lungs, and related blood vessels and arteries.

Compound set Performing two different exercises for the same primary muscle group in succession without a period of rest in between.

Concentric contraction The shortening of a muscle against resistance in order to create action in a joint. For example, if you want to bring your hand toward your shoulder, you bend your elbow, and thereby flex your biceps muscles. As you do this, the biceps muscles contract concentrically.

Cross-training Combining a variety of activities into a workout program to ward off overuse injuries, train the muscles in a well-rounded manner, and prevent boredom.

Delayed onset muscle soreness (DOMS) Normal soreness that occurs after engaging in an activity that your body is not accustomed to; DOMS may develop up to 12 hours after a workout and usually lasts for a day or two before gradually subsiding. DOMS is thought to be caused by microscopic tears and swelling around muscle fibers. Warming up and cooling down will minimize soreness, as will avoiding taking on too much, too soon.

Deltoids The muscles of the shoulders. The anterior deltoids are the muscles at the front of the shoulders, the medial deltoids are on the sides, and the posterior deltoids are in the rear.

Dynamic stretching Moving parts of your body in smooth, controlled, and gradual motions in order to increase the range of motion to its natural limit. An example of a dynamic stretch is a slow and controlled torso twist.

Eccentric contraction Pronounced E-SEN-TRIC, not EK-CENT-TRIK, this is the lengthening of a weight-loaded muscle.

Electrolytes Minerals such as sodium, potassium, and magnesium that help keep the fluids of the body in a balanced state. Along with water, these minerals are lost through perspiration. Sports drinks are an effective way to replenish lost electrolytes.

Endorphins Biochemical compounds in the brain that are released during periods of extended and continuous exercise. Endorphins are natural pain relievers and contribute to feelings of exercise-induced euphoria, such as the "runner's high."

Extension Movement at a joint that increases the angle between the two bones it connects. For example, a knee extension is performed by moving the shin bone (front of lower leg) away from the femur (back of thigh).

Flexion Bending a joint to decrease the angle between the two bones it connects. For example, a knee flexion is performed by moving the shin bone (front of lower leg) toward the femur (back of thigh).

Flexibility The range of motion around a joint or series of joints.

Functional training Training with the goal of increasing strength, improving coordination, and enhancing overall efficiency in activities that simulate real-life actions.

Gluteals An all-encompassing term for the three muscles of the rear end, the gluteus maximus, the gluteus medius, and the gluteus minimus.

Hamstrings A group of three muscles located in the backs of the thighs that originate around the pelvic bone and extend below the knee.

GLOSSARY

High impact Activities that are jarring to the joints.

Iliotibial band (IT band) A band of thick fibrous tissue that runs down the outside of the leg, beginning at the hip and extending to just below the knee joint. It works in conjunction with several muscles in the thigh to stabilize the knee joint.

Isometric exercise When a muscle generates a steady force against a resistance without overcoming it. There is no movement involved in such an exercise.

Kinesiology Derived from the Greek words *kinein*, "to move," and *logos*, "to study." Kinesiology is the science of human movement.

Latissimus dorsi (lats) The largest muscles of the back, which create the sculpted V-shape at the sides of the body.

Load The amount of weight designated for an exercise.

Low impact Low-impact aerobic exercise was introduced at the IDEA Health and Fitness Association's annual conference in 1985, offering a remedy for injuries caused by joint-jarring high-impact exercises. At the time, low-impact aerobics was defined as exercise that maintained one foot on the ground at all times. Today, the term refers to any exercise that is not jarring to the joints.

Metabolism The rate at which your body converts nutrients and other substances into energy. The speed of your metabolism affects how quickly (or slowly) your body burns calories no matter what you are doing—running a marathon, working at your desk, or sleeping.

Muscle failure A muscle's temporary inability to contract fully as a result of high-intensity exertion. For example, if you've done 30 push-ups and feel you absolutely can't do one more without a break, you've reached muscle failure.

One rep max The greatest amount of weight that can be lifted with proper form for a maximum of one repetition.

Osteoporosis A condition characterized by decreased bone mass. Weight-bearing and resistance training exercises help keep bones strong and can prevent the development of osteoporosis.

Overtraining A technical term for the condition brought on by too much training and/or too little rest. This is usually characterized by injury, illness, and/or decreased exercise capacity.

Pectorals (pecs) The pectoralis major and the pectoralis minor are the two pairs of muscles of the chest.

Periodization Systematic process of planning variations into a resistance training program over the course of weeks, months, or a year, in order to maximize results.

Plyometric exercise A type of training that helps develop fast-twitch muscle fibers, and increases explosive athletic power. Plyometric exercises work to help the muscles develop the ability to rapidly and vigorously lengthen and recoil.

PNF stretching This stands for "proprioceptive neuromuscular facilitation" and was initially developed as a method of rehabilitating stroke victims. This stretching technique combines passive and isometric stretching.

Prone Lying face down or on your stomach.

Proprioception The body's ability to sense its spacial position, location, orientation, and movement.

Quadriceps (quads) The four muscles of the front part of the thigh: the vastus intermedius, the vastus lateralis, the vastus medialis, and the rectus femoris.

Rate of perceived exertion (RPE) This scale, developed by Gunner Borg in 1998, associates a range of sensations with numbers in order to help identify levels of intensity during an activity.

Reps The number of times weight is lifted and lowered within a given exercise.

Sanskrit One of the oldest languages known to human beings. It is the classical language of India, and the language of yoga.

Sets A group of exercise repetitions performed in succession.

Spot To act as a safety net and/or offer minor assistance to someone lifting a weight. A spotter keeps a close eye on the lifter, helping guide movements and offering assistance if necessary.

Static stretching Stretching a group of muscles to their farthest point within a given range of motion and maintaining that position.

Strip set Performing a set beginning with a heavy weight and moving to lighter weights upon reaching muscle failure with no period of rest in between.

Superset Performing two exercises for opposing muscle groups in succession without a period of rest in between.

Supine Lying face up or on your back.

Threshold (also known as *Lactate threshold* or *Anaerobic threshold*) Exercise at a level of intensity that causes lactic acid to build up in the muscles more quickly than the body is able to process it. At this intensity, carbohydrates become the muscles' major source of energy, and the supply of oxygen available to them begins to fall.

Triceps The triceps muscles, or triceps brachii, extend the forearm at the elbow and function as supporting muscles for pushing exercises that target muscles of the chest.

Unilateral Working one side of the body at a time. Unilateral training is used to help create a balance in strength on both sides of the body.

Warm-up Low intensity movement that prepares the body for more demanding activities or exercise by stimulating blood flow through the muscles and raising the temperature of the body.

Weight-bearing exercise Exercises that require muscles to work against gravity in order to support the body's weight with or without additional weight. A few examples are stair climbing, hiking, running, and weight lifting. Such exercises are known for helping to build denser, stronger bones.

"Working-in" To alternate using a piece of equipment with a fellow gym member in between sets.

INDEX

INDEX

ABOUT THE AUTHORS

Gregg Cook is a national fitness educator with eight years of modern dance and movement training and an additional decade of experience in the fitness industry. With an avid following in New York City, Gregg is recognized by *New York Magazine* as one of the city's elite fitness instructors. He is a BOSU, Urban Rebounding, Body Bar, and Schwinn Indoor Cycling master trainer, and his extensive work as a program developer include his signature TerraCycle, Body Bar Blast, and RE-Circuit classes. Gregg teaches at Equinox Fitness Clubs throughout New York City, is a national spokesperson for Amino Vital, an amino acid-based sports drink, and runs a private personal training, coaching, and consulting business. He is regularly featured as a fitness expert in national press and on television, including such programs as *Today* and *Good Morning America*.

Fatima d'Almeida-Cook is a native New Yorker and fitness devotee. She is an accomplished writer about lifestyle and fitness issues.

Both authors have also written *Body Bar: 133 Moves for Full-Body Fitness*, published by Sterling Publishing.

PHOTO CREDITS

Explanation of abbreviations: b = bottom of page, c = center of page, l = left column, r = right column, t = top of page

Courtesy of Body Bar Systems, Inc.: 174 (r)

Courtesy of Body Wedge 21: 174 (l)

Courtesy of BOSU: 167 (l)

Courtesy of Concept 2, Inc.: 159 (r)

Courtesy of Cybex International Inc.: 134 (c), 136 (r), 137 (b), 144, 145, 147 (t), 149 (t, b), 158

Courtesy of Heart Rate, Inc.: 159 (l)

Courtesy of Nautilus Inc.: 131(r), 132, 133 (l, r), 134 (t, b), 135, 137 (t), 138, 139, 140 (l, r), 141 (l), 142, 143 (l, r), 146 (l, r), 147 (b), 148 (l, r), 153, 154 (l, r), 155, 156, 160, 167 (r), 168, 170 (r), 173 (t)

Courtesy of Perform Better, Inc.: 149 (c), 165 (r), 166 (r), 175 (t, b), 179 (l)

Courtesy of Power Systems, Inc.: 163, 164 (b), 165 (l), 166 (l), 171 (l), 176 (b), 177

Courtesy of Precor USA: 131 (l), 141 (r), 175 (b), 179 (r)

Courtesy of ShutterStock: 2, 8, 14, 24, 32, 58, 126, 150, 180, 216

Courtesy of ThinkFit: 173 (c)

Courtesy of Urban Rebounding: 170 (l)